The Ultimate guide to Fitness

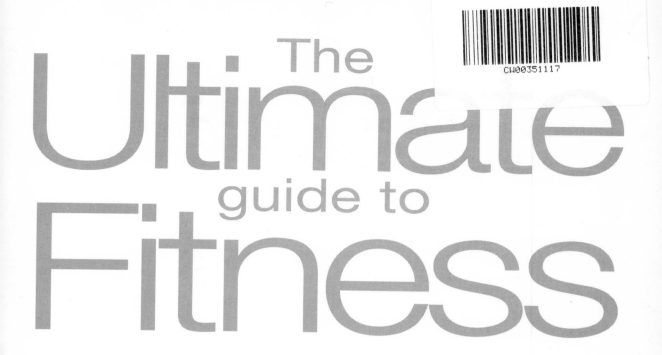

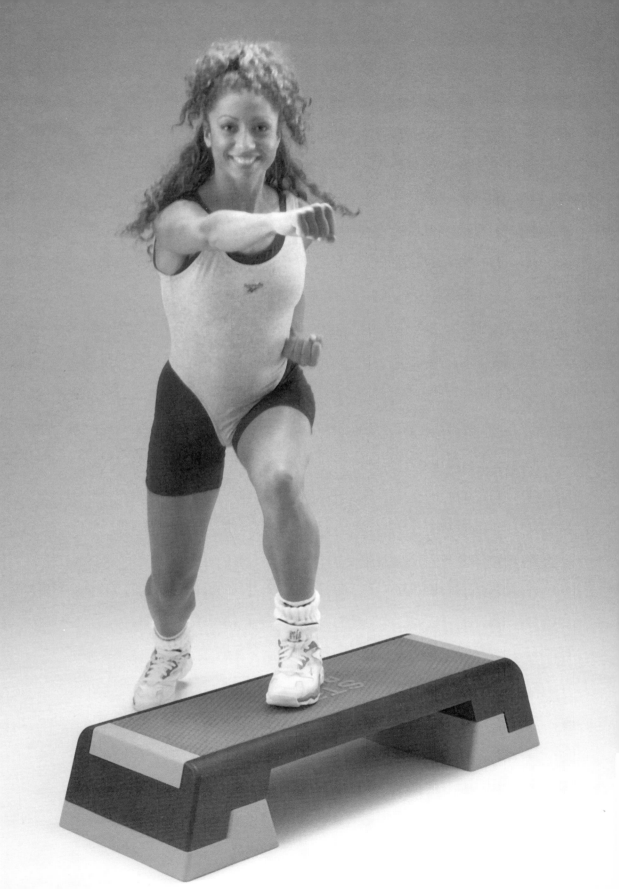

The Ultimate guide to Fitness

Chantal Gosselin

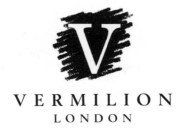

VERMILION
LONDON

*To Edith and René for my humour
and healthy attitude to life.*

First published in 1995
1 3 5 7 9 10 8 6 4 2

First published in the United Kingdom in 1995 by Vermilion an imprint of Ebury Press
Random House, 20 Vauxhall Bridge Road, London SW1V 2SA

Random House Australia (Pty) Limited
20 Alfred Street, Milsons Point, Sydney, New South Wales 2061, Australia

Random House New Zealand Limited
18 Poland Road, Glenfield, Auckland 10, New Zealand

Random House South Africa (Pty) Limited PO Box 337, Bergvlei, South Africa

Random House UK Limited Reg. No. 954009

Editor: Jan Bowmer Design: Jerry Goldie Graphic Design
Photography: Jon Stewart Cover photograph by Mike Henderson

Exercises demonstrated by Lisa Brockwell and Dean Hodgkin

A CIP catalogue record for this book is available from the British Library
ISBN 0-09-178370-4

Printed and bound in Great Britain by Clays Ltd, St Ives plc

Warning

Prior to commencing any exercise programme, you should first consult
your physician. If you have a medical condition or are pregnant, the
exercises in this book should not be followed without first consulting
your doctor. All guidelines and warnings should be read carefully, and
the author and publisher cannot accept responsibility for injuries or
damage arising out of a failure to comply with the same.

Contents

Acknowledgments

Thanks to Lorna L. Francis, Ph.D., who is involved in educational programme development for Reebok University and who is currently a consultant for the California Governor's Council on Physical Fitness and Sport.

Thanks also to the following UK experts for their advice and guidance: Anita Bean, B.Sc., nutritionist, for advising on nutrition; Pat Dunn, BA, M.Sc., chartered psychologist, for advising on social and emotional health; Adrianne Hardman, Ph.D., Senior Lecturer at the Department of Physical Education, Sports Sciences and Recreation Management at Loughborough University, for advising on exercise physiology; Neil Armstrong, Ph.D., FRSM, F.I.Biol., Professor of Health and Exercise Sciences at Exeter University and President of the Physical Education Association of Great Britain and Northern Ireland; Mike Kelly, B.Sc., M.Sc., Ph.D., Reader in Health Sciences at Leeds Metropolitan University; Patrick Squire BA, MA, Senior Lecturer in Exercise and Health at the Moray House Institute, Edinburgh.

Finally, thanks to Diana Moran and Larry Mitchell for their continued support.

Introduction

Back in the early eighties Reebok designed the very first aerobics sports shoe. To be able to do this successfully, it was necessary to understand aerobics thoroughly. From those early days through to today Reebok has placed great importance on working with some of the world's top fitness experts to pioneer a series of innovative fitness programmes that help educate the instructor and offer the public new and enjoyable ways of exercising. Consequently, Reebok is renowned as a leading authority on fitness and athletics training.

These fitness programmes are now pooled under one umbrella, known as Reebok University. Launched in 1993, Reebok University fulfilled a long-standing vision of Reebok International: to establish a 'university without walls', offering quality-researched, state-of-the-art sports and fitness programming, education and publishing for industry professionals and participants throughout the world.

Reebok was one of the first organizations to research a fitness programme before releasing it to the professional instructor or the general public. In 1989 it created the new trend in step aerobics with the launch of its Step Reebok® programme. Since then, all subsequent Reebok University exercise programmes undergo research and scrutiny by specialist development teams and experts around the world before being published and are taught worldwide by a team of specially trained instructors.

Reebok's philosophy has always been one of education: education to prevent injury; to encourage sports and fitness participation at all levels; to promote better and more innovative teaching and enhanced performance, be it five-a-side soccer (now an international event), tennis star training camps for youngsters or pre-season conditioning programmes for athletes.

Regular exercise is a must if we are to measure up to the stresses and strains of modern living. Everyone can exercise, but it must be enjoyable, it must be the right type of exercise and it must fit in with our lifestyle or we won't keep it up. The aim of *The Ultimate Guide to Fitness*, therefore, is to show how you can achieve a regularly active lifestyle – one that suits your mood and your personality.

How to Use this Book

This book is divided into three parts. Part One explains the benefits of exercise, how the body works and what total fitness entails, as well as dispelling some common myths.

Part Two outlines the basic principles that need to be followed in order for fitness to be effective. It offers a step-by-step plan that helps you assess your current fitness level and determine which type of exercise programme would suit you best, plus guidelines on planning your own schedule of exercise, from getting started through to injury prevention and proper technique.

Part Three contains the Reebok University training programmes, plus a basic workout for complete beginners. Advice is given on the correct way to warm up and cool down and the proper technique for each specific workout. There are tips on how to keep going once you've started your new and active lifestyle – how to maintain your willpower and enthusiasm. It also looks at other lifestyle habits that affect your health and wellbeing.

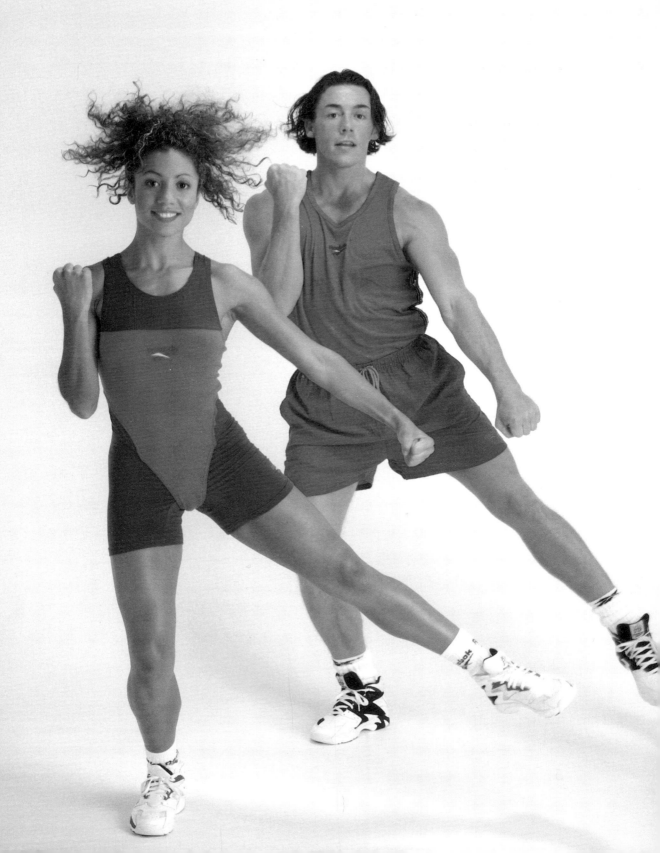

Part One

Why Exercise?

Our bodies are essentially designed to cope with a certain level of physical activity. Until recent times a fair amount of that physical activity formed part of our everyday lives. Fulfilling our basic needs for food and water and having to travel about or defend ourselves provided regular physical challenges.

In ancient times, not being able to walk or run meant that we would have either starved or were likely to have been killed by an enemy tribe or wild animals. Now that we live in an automated era, much of the physical activity necessary for everyday survival is already done for us, and the nearest most of us get to being a hunter/gatherer is a trip to the local supermarket or a weekend's fishing!

So, in order to keep our bodies tuned and functioning efficiently we have to make a concerted effort to be active. With all the mental effort demanded of us in keeping our working, family or social lives together, that extra push we need to get us up off the sofa and out of the door to walk the dog is, for many of us, just too difficult to summon up.

Often, it's not until we find ourselves confronted with a major illness or find ourselves averting our eyes from the full-length mirror on the bathroom wall that many of us start to seriously consider the state that our bodies are in and our level of fitness.

What Exercise Can Do For You

Regular exercise is important for everyone. Yes, you have probably heard that a million times, but have you thought what this actually means in terms of your own health?

It is now widely accepted that prevention is better than cure, and in recent years we have seen an increasing popularity in the GP referrals' system. This is where doctors work together with local health clubs or fitness experts to plan specific programmes of regular exercise for individual patients to help deal with ailments such as heart disease or simply to improve patients' fitness levels.

But, as well as rehabilitate, exercise can contribute greatly to lessening the risk or even help in the control of many illnesses.

Exercise for Health

Research into exercise continues in many major universities across the world. We now know that a regular planned programme of exercise can help

✦ Reduce the risk of heart disease
✦ Lower blood pressure levels
✦ Improve cholesterol levels
✦ Lessen the risk of osteoporosis
✦ Control asthma
✦ Control adult-onset diabetes
✦ Promote weight loss
✦ Manage stress
✦ Delay breathlessness
✦ Improve the blood circulation system
✦ Improve the functioning of the heart
✦ Improve postural problems
✦ Improve agility, balance and flexibility
✦ Improve strength
✦ Improve our sense of wellbeing.

Different types of exercise can help specific conditions. For example, regular and repetitive weight-bearing exercise such as fitness walking can prove extremely beneficial for pre-menopausal women in reducing their risk of suffering osteoporosis in later life. Regular aerobic exercise can improve the working of the cardiorespiratory (heart and lungs) system. Everyone can benefit from regular exercise taken at a moderate level and, while we don't all have to become Olympic athletes overnight, we ought to be aware of the dangers of inadequate exercise and diet.

What Does Fitness Mean?

To some people 'fitness' means not being ill, while to others it's a question of how long it takes them to complete a marathon.

For the elderly it could mean the difference between independence and dependence. However, due to extensive research into all areas of health and exercise, it is now possible to assess an individual's level of fitness and design an appropriate exercise programme to suit their specific needs. But it's important to remember that fitness levels are relative to the individual. What may be a good level of fitness for one person may not always be right for another, hence the term 'personal fitness'. Everyone can benefit from leading a more active lifestyle and in doing so increase his or her personal fitness level.

What Constitutes Total Fitness?

Total fitness is made up of several components. To evaluate your total fitness you need to consider your physical, mental, and nutritional health status and your social and emotional skills management. All these factors have a significant effect on each other and contribute to your overall wellbeing.

For instance, your overall health benefits will be greater if, in addition to taking up regular exercise, you also monitor your diet and give up smoking. But, equally, to fanatically embark on a strenuous exercise routine that leaves little time for other areas of your life could just be a mask for more serious emotional problems which would only become worse if ignored.

Fitness assessments (see page 36) carried out by most gyms and health clubs will only evaluate certain physical attributes.

Entirely separate specialist skills are required for dealing with both nutritional or eating disorders and emotional wear and tear (the appropriate specialist can be contacted via your GP).

The Physical Components of Fitness

The physical components of fitness fall into two main categories. The first, *health-related fitness*, relates to the factors that affect your health and wellbeing, and this is what most fitness training programmes are concerned with. The second, *skill-related fitness*, relates to the skill-building factors which are often the focus of sports training programmes.

Physical Fitness Components

Health-related Fitness	Skill-related Fitness
Body composition	Agility
Cardiovascular endurance	Balance
Flexibility	Coordination
Muscular endurance	Power
Muscular strength	Reaction time
	Speed

Health-related Components: What They Mean

Body composition is the term used to describe the ratio of fat to lean body mass (i.e. everything that is not fat, including bone and muscle). This is not to be confused with body weight, which is the total weight of the entire body. By using universal guidelines, it is possible to measure body composition to determine the level of fat on the body, which is an important factor in health care. Body composition can be measured by your GP or a health-care professional.

Cardiovascular endurance or aerobic fitness is the ability to maintain at least a moderate level of activity using the large muscles of the body (e.g. swimming, running, brisk walking) for a period of time – usually a minimum of 15 to 20 minutes – long enough to produce beneficial changes to the heart, lungs and circulatory system. The healthier and more efficient the heart, lungs and associated blood vessels, the easier it is for the individual to achieve even the minimum level of aerobic fitness.

Factfile

A recent survey in the UK revealed a clear association between an inactive lifestyle and chronic disease, plus an increased risk of stroke and ischaemic (lack of blood supply) heart disease in inactive, overweight middle-aged men (Allied Dunbar National Fitness Survey, England, 1992).

Flexibility is how much range of movement an individual has in each of the joints. Having appropriate flexibility enables you to perform everyday activities safely and efficiently, e.g. touching your toes, reaching for the top shelf, pulling up the zip at the back of your dress.

Muscular endurance is the capacity of a muscle or a group of muscles to maintain or repeat a movement for a set period of time without getting tired, e.g. how long it takes before your arms tire when you are vacuuming the stairs.

Muscular strength is the amount of force exerted by a muscle or a group of muscles, e.g. how much weight you can lift or push. Muscular strength is not necessarily equal throughout the body. For instance, the arms may be weaker than the legs, or one arm may be stronger than the other.

Skill-related Components: What They Mean

Agility is the ability to rapidly change direction or weight distribution (e.g. moving from foot to foot) while retaining control and is dependent on speed, balance and coordination, e.g. moving about easily, reaching, bending, twisting or turning while cleaning the house or chasing the dog.

Balance is the ability to move about or stand still without swaying, stumbling or falling over.

Coordination is the ability to perform a sequence of a range of movements accurately, rhythmically and with appropriate timing, e.g. continuously hitting a ball with a racket as in tennis or squash.

Power is the ability to perform an action with both strength and speed, e.g. being able to swing a bat or racket with force and speed.

Reaction time is the ability to select and decide quickly on a physical response, e.g. jumping back from the road as a vehicle splashes through a puddle.

Speed is the ability to move as fast as possible, e.g. running.

It's All Trainable

The components of fitness are very much like the components of a car. The better the condition we keep them in and the more protection we give them, the better their performance.

All of the above fitness components are to a greater or lesser extent trainable – in other words, we can improve each of them through a certain amount of regular exercise.

A balanced exercise programme aimed at improving all-round fitness should include each of the above health-related fitness components. A sports-oriented programme, where the aim is to improve a player's skill at that particular sport or group of sports, is more likely to focus on the skill-related factors.

However, the two categories can overlap. In an all-round fitness programme certain skills are bound to improve as a by-product of the workout. For example, the main focus of an aerobics dance class is cardiovascular conditioning, yet the nature of the activity – rhythmic movement to music – involves a certain amount of agility and coordination. Equally, a sports-oriented programme will also improve aspects of health-related fitness as a result of the physical activity involved in the sports-type skill drills. The greatest improvements, however, will occur in the aspects that are focused on most frequently.

We Are What We Do

The more fitness training we do, the more physical skills we will develop along the way and, equally, the more sports we play, the more we will hone our skills and increase our level of fitness. This is what the experts call *specificity training*, which means that people who, for example, do strength training will get stronger, people who run will improve their cardiovascular

> **Factfile**
>
> Our parents and grandparents were from a much more active era. In the early 1930s Mary Bagot Stack set up the Women's League of Health and Beauty, which was designed to encourage women of all social classes to take up movement to music for their own health benefit. At that time, it was considered a 'controversial' organization, yet it attracted some 250 thousand members throughout Europe.

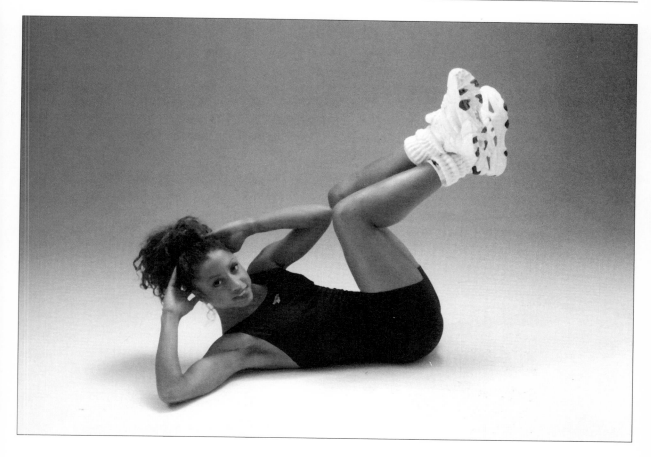

attributes etc. Specific adaptations are caused by specifically induced demands.

As we develop specific skills from frequently playing a specific sport or carrying out a specific activity, at the same time we will also develop specific fitness benefits. For example, body-builders who regularly lift heavy weights will become very good at lifting heavy weights because they will train their muscular strength, but they may not be able to run very far or for very long and therefore have poor cardiovascular fitness. Equally, marathon runners who are 'aerobically' fit as a result of regularly running long distances may not have much muscular strength and therefore not be able to lift a great weight. Furthermore, marathon runners won't necessarily be comfortable with short sprints, because their muscles will have trained to cope with running long distances.

On the positive side, our bodies generally respond well to exercise – indeed they thrive on it – and adapt to new challenges very quickly, which is why it is important when planning an exercise programme always to start at the level that is right for our ability and to progress at a suitable rate that keeps both our minds and our bodies interested.

While running a marathon or entering the next Olympics or even the local tennis tournament may not be on your personal agenda, improving the quality of life and making the daily grind less of a grind ought to be on everyone's.

Regular exercise may not turn you into an overnight star of track or field, but it should enhance your ability to do the things you either have to do or want to do.

The Body in Action

Mention the words anatomy and physiology, and most people assume they are going to be blinded by science. But being aware of what happens within our bodies on a day-to-day basis is important in understanding why we all need some level of exercise. It will also help ensure we select the right exercise programme and help prevent exercise mistakes or injury.

The Human Structure

Think of the human body as being structured like a puppet. The wooden arms and legs of the puppet resemble the human skeleton, with 'bones' connected at certain points by hinge-like joints. And the strings that the puppeteer uses to make the puppet move, work in much the same way as our muscles.

The puppeteer in our case is the brain and vital organs, which bring to life the otherwise lifeless puppet.

The Bones

There are some 206 bones in the human skeleton and they have two main functions. The first is to form the mechanical scaffolding of the body (without them we would be like rag dolls) and provide somewhere for muscles to attach themselves. The second is to act as protection for our vital organs such as the brain, the heart, lungs and spinal cord.

The bones in our bodies are as alive as we are and are kept healthy by the blood-supply system, which feeds bone-developing cells located within the bone.

At birth our bones are soft and flexible. Throughout childhood our bones develop, gradually laying down more calcium which eventually causes our bones to become hard.

In adulthood our bones become a lot harder, reaching a peak in bone mass between the ages of 20 and 30.

From about the age of 35 there is a natural bone loss in both men and women which speeds up with age and peaks dramatically around the age of 50. This process tends to occur more rapidly in women in the first five to ten years following the menopause because of the decreases in oestrogen levels. The loss of calcium from our bones causes them to become progressively weaker, and in old age they can become very brittle and vulnerable to fracturing, particularly in post-menopausal women. This brittle-bone condition is known in medical circles as osteopenia, which leads to the disease commonly known as osteoporosis, where even a slight knock can easily cause the bones to fracture.

Osteoporosis is now considered a life-threatening disease, mainly because a series of fractures experienced by an elderly person can often lead to complications such as pneumonia and bring about premature death. At the very least, it can lead to severe disability causing much hardship and unhappiness both to sufferers and their families.

Sadly, osteoporosis is on the increase and the elderly are more prone to this condition than ever before because they are living longer and less actively and eating a less nutritious diet. Although research is constantly being done, it is still not known why certain women seem to be more prone to this disease than others. However, you are more likely to be at risk of osteoporosis if any of the following apply to you:

✦ Osteoporosis is common in the family
✦ You are or have been a heavy smoker
✦ You have a high intake of alcohol or caffeine
✦ You are or have been underweight for long periods of time or anorexic
✦ You have an early menopause
✦ Your diet is poor, too low in calcium, or too high in protein
✦ You are inactive (whether a couch potato or invalid)
✦ You have had cortisone and thyroid treatments.

Bones and Exercise

Research has shown that regular exercise, particularly in the bone-forming years during childhood can strengthen bones. Maintaining a regular programme of weight-bearing (sometimes called bone-loading) exercise can slow down bone loss and increase bone density.

Therefore, it's important to include activities such as fitness walking, running, aerobics, weight-training, stair climbing or step training in your exercise programme each week. While improvements can still be made in old age, the most important time to improve bone health is when you are young. Young adults can help prevent bone brittleness in old age by exercising now – but it needs to be kept up for life!

If you already suffer from osteoporosis, please check with your GP before starting any new exercise regime.

The Joints

A joint is the point where two bones meet, usually a place where the body needs a certain amount of controlled movement. For example, imagine trying to walk without knee joints. You would have to use a swaying side-to-side action to move each foot forward and this would put a tremendous strain on the back. So, the knee joints are there to allow the legs to bend and the feet to swing through for walking or running purposes.

There are three types of joints:

1 Mobile (or moveable) as in the knee, hip or shoulder.
2 Slightly mobile as in the spine.
3 Immobile (unmoveable) as in the skull or breastbone.

Some joints need to be strong and some need to be moveable, depending on the job they have to do. The more moveable a joint, the weaker and more vulnerable to injury it tends to be. Each joint has its own natural protective equipment in the form of cartilage and fibrous tissue, fluid sacs and ligaments, all of which is designed to keep the joint functioning properly. However, joints still need to be treated with respect just like any mechanical part.

Factfile

✦ **Some 50 per cent of women have osteoporosis in the ten-year period following menopause, increasing to some 70 per cent in the subsequent ten years.**

✦ **Men suffer from osteoporosis too, although the condition is not quite so severe as with women, and only one out of every 12 men over the age of 70 shows symptoms.**

✦ **Caucasian women are more prone to osteoporosis than women of African origin.**

Factfile

✦ **Individuals with a history of regular and continued sport or exercise participation tend to have better bone health in old age.**

✦ **Regular weight-bearing exercise strengthens bones.**

✦ **Using correct posture and technique protects joints.**

✦ **Exercise keeps joints resilient and mobile.**

The Muscles

The main function of muscle is to keep the body working and moving. Muscle falls into three types: voluntary, involuntary and cardiac.

Voluntary Muscles

The voluntary group of muscles is the largest group and is also known as skeletal muscle (the muscles just underneath the skin and which are clearly defined in athletes with highly toned bodies). Skeletal muscle moulds the flesh and much of the outer shape of the body. Like the strings on the puppet we mentioned earlier, the main function of skeletal or voluntary muscle is to defy gravity by holding us upright and enabling us to move our bones/bodies about.

> ### Factfile
> ✦ **There are more than 650 muscles in the body.**
> ✦ **Muscles account for some 35– 45 per cent of total body**

Skeletal muscles can either be very large, like the muscles in the thighs, buttocks or back, or they can be tiny, like those in the eyes.

The skeletal muscle responds to specific orders from the brain, in response to signals received via our sensors (eyes, ears, nose, skin), and delivered via the neuromuscular or nervous system.

Most skeletal muscle joins one bone to another. One end of the muscle is attached to an immobile section of bone for stability, and the other end is attached to a bone that needs to move.

Muscles usually work by contracting and relaxing, either by being lengthened (stretched) – these are known as eccentric contractions – or shortened (concentric contractions) to enable the joints to move.

However, muscles can still work without any joint movement being involved, and this is called an isometric (or equal length) contraction. This is what happens, for instance, when you are carrying heavy shopping bags and your elbows remain in the same position.

Pairing up

Most muscles work in pairs, so while one muscle is shortening in order to bend a limb, another muscle (usually on the opposite side of the limb) is being lengthened (stretched) to allow the related joint to move. For example, a very rough description of what happens when you walk is that the muscles at the back of your thigh (hamstrings) shorten and, at the same time, the muscles at the front of the thigh (quadriceps) lengthen to allow the knee to bend. To straighten out the knee, the quadriceps will then shorten and the hamstrings will lengthen to allow the knee joint to extend.

Stabilizers

Finally, the skeletal muscles can also act as stabilizers during certain actions. For example, try standing on one leg and lifting the other. Now, feel the muscles in the thigh and buttock of your standing leg. They will have instantly tightened up to support your whole body while the other leg is off the floor. Isn't it amazing how quickly and efficiently they work? Just imagine, your legs do that to a greater or lesser degree each time you walk. Different muscles will automatically come into action as you change either the gradient that you walk on or the speed, or if you add an arm swing as you walk.

Involuntary and Cardiac Muscles

These two muscle types are essentially involved with our vital organs. *Involuntary* muscles (such as the muscles in the digestive system) are on a permanent 'standing order' controlled by the brain which can't be interrupted except by certain medications or death itself. The *cardiac* muscle is the heart. Yes, the heart is a muscle, and regular vigorous exercise will help the heart function more efficiently. In other words, the fitter the heart, the better it copes with its everyday workload. A fit heart does not have to beat as frequently as an unfit one, since it is able to push more blood out each time it pumps. Again, the heart acts on orders directly from the brain and keeps constantly beating to pump blood around the body until the heart's blood supply is restricted or until it becomes worn out through age.

Muscles and Exercise

Muscles are made up of lots of fibres. For muscles to be firm and healthy these muscle fibres need to be given sufficient work. Exercise therefore stimulates the muscle fibres. The more work the muscles do, the more oxygen they require and this is supplied via the blood. The bigger muscles, or major muscle groups as they are sometimes called (the muscles in the buttocks, thighs, back and shoulders), require even more oxygen than smaller muscles when being worked and, accordingly, require a greater blood supply. This is why when we exercise these major muscle groups our heart rate and breathing rate increase.

> **Factfile**
>
> A simple act such as walking involves nearly all of your muscles. The abdominal (stomach) and back muscles are busy holding the spine and head and shoulders up and allowing your trunk to twist slightly and your arms to work in opposition to your legs (i.e. as your left leg swings forward, so does the right arm – hopefully!).

Muscle tone

To maintain muscle tone and firmness, the muscles have to be exercised regularly. And since muscles quickly become accustomed to exercise, the challenge needs to be gradually increased (see page 24) in order to see further benefits.

Working out with weights

It is a very common misunderstanding that women who work out with weights (resistance training) will build huge muscles.

Muscle-building is largely dependent on a substantial presence of the male hormone testosterone. Most men have a good natural dose of it in their bodies while women have only a small amount – just enough for them to be able to build sufficient muscle for their needs. Therefore, for the average woman, a programme of light but frequent resistance exercise should do no more than lift and tone the areas of the body she wants to lift and tone.

To build the kind of muscle sported by professional body-builders it would be necessary to lift enormous amounts of weights and train gruelling hours. Light-weight training with lots of repetitions (but generally not exceeding 20 repetitions per exercise), however, will help build a more natural body shape, one that is toned but not bulky. Many top tennis players, swimmers and athletes train with weights to help improve their sports performance, yet they remain relatively slender.

Muscle soreness

Skeletal muscle soreness is usually the result of doing too much too soon, taking up a new form of exercise, or diving into a strenuous bout of exercise, especially if you have not warmed up and cooled down properly.

When a muscle is being exercised it produces waste products. If we exercise too severely or do a new form of exercise, the muscle fibres will not be accustomed to this particular demand, and waste products can therefore build up in the muscle. This build-up can result in muscle soreness within 24 to 48 hours after exercising. The soreness should slowly diminish over the following two or three days. A proper cool-down and stretch session will help reduce the risk of soreness.

> **Factfile**
>
> + Muscles can be made firmer with exercise.
> + Your heart is a muscle – regular exercise makes it function more efficiently.
> + Most women won't develop big muscles from exercising with weights.
> + Healthy trained muscle burns more calories.
> + Weak muscles leave the joints at a higher risk of injury.

Muscle reduction

Muscle bulk can be reduced by illness or old age. Anyone who has ever broken a leg will have experienced a withering of the muscles in that leg. Once the injury has healed, these muscles will then need to be built up again. Equally, if an individual is bedridden for a period of time, the body's muscle tone and mass will diminish, and it will be necessary to spend time on gently and slowly rebuilding the muscle before starting or resuming an exercise programme.

It's important never to exercise when you are ill or just recovering from illness. Always complete a full convalescent period before resuming exercise.

The Vital Organs

Regular exercise can have a positive effect on our internal organs, mainly because an active lifestyle means more oxygen and less fat in the body's systems, which improves the quality of the blood supply to all our vital working parts. The two systems that are most directly involved in exercise are the heart and blood circulatory system and the lungs or respiratory system.

The Heart and Lungs

The heart weighs about three-quarters of a pound and is a continuously working muscle with a dual pumping system. The lungs work like a pair of bellows drawing in oxygen from the air and exhaling carbon dioxide through the nose and mouth.

The two work very closely together in circulating and cleansing the blood. The heart receives blood filled with oxygen (oxygenated) from the lungs, then pumps it out to all parts of the body via the arteries. The blood flows through the veins and back to the heart, which then pumps this used blood into the lungs and, thus, the cycle begins again.

The heartbeat

It's this pumping action that forms the heartbeat. When the body starts to exercise, the muscles involved require more blood, and so the heart beats faster to increase the supply. The fitter a heart, the more blood it can push out in each pump, and therefore does not need to beat as frequently. This is why the heart of a fit person is well equipped to cope with everyday demands as well as physical or emotional pressure.

The pulse rate

The pulse rate (heart rate) is an indication of how hard the heart is working, and can be a useful guide to an individual's fitness level (see page 26).

Your pulse rate varies throughout the day according to your temperament, lifestyle, diet, frame of mind and fitness level. It is at its lowest first thing in the morning when you wake up but before you get out of bed. This is called the *resting heart rate* and, generally speaking, in the case of adults the lower this is, the better. The *maximum heart rate* is the maximum number of times the heart can beat per minute.

The pulse rate can also give an indication of the state of an individual's health, which is why doctors take the pulse rate of patients to check if they fall within the normal levels. On average the heart beats about 70 to 80 times a minute in a healthy adult, although this can vary according to sex, build, age and level of fitness.

A very fit individual will tend to have a slightly lower resting pulse rate – say between 50 and 60 beats per minute (bpm) — whereas a seriously unfit individual may have a resting pulse rate of 70 to 90 beats per minute or higher.

But before you rush off to the doctor to have your pulse rate checked, there are several perfectly normal factors that can affect your regular heartbeat. These include

- ✦ coffee, alcohol or other stimulants
- ✦ having just eaten a meal
- ✦ having just walked up a hill or a flight of stairs
- ✦ having had an argument or heated conversation
- ✦ stressful situations such as waiting for a bus when you're in a hurry
- ✦ worrying or feeling ill with a cold or minor illness.

People who have a very high or very low resting heart rate should always check with their doctor before beginning any form of exercise programme. Registering an unusually high heart rate when you are not exercising can be a sign of high blood pressure or illness and should always be investigated medically. But the good news is that regular aerobic exercise can lower the daily heart rate and make the heart pump more efficiently.

Regular exercise is now prescribed by many doctors for the rehabilitation of cardiac patients (those recovering from heart surgery), for lowering blood pressure and for reducing the risk of recurrent heart attack. Eighty-five per cent of patients who have undergone heart surgery take up the opportunity of exercising regularly under supervision.

Factfile

- ✦ **The maximum number of times the heart can beat per minute is approximately 220.**
- ✦ **The maximum heart rate reduces by one beat for every year of age. Therefore, in the case of a 20-year-old, the maximum number of times the heart can beat in one minute is approximately 200.**
- ✦ **During exercise, the heart rate increases and can go up to as high as 180–200 beats per minute.**
- ✦ **In a fit person the heart rate will not increase too rapidly or go too high and, most importantly, will drop back down to its normal level fairly quickly after exercise.**

Blood Circulation

Blood is vital to our bodies and is literally the lifeblood of the human structure. Blood supplies all our vital organs, muscles, bones and even our skin with nutrients and oxygen by means of the arteries – the major network of blood-carrying pipes. Having delivered its load of nutrients and oxygen, the blood flows back to the heart, carrying the waste products offloaded by exercising muscles. These waste products are then disposed of by being expired (breathed out) through the lungs.

Healthy Blood

Because of the important role that veins and arteries play in this delivery-and-return process, it is vital that they stay healthy and able to function. A blockage in the circulatory network will put extra demands on the heart which, in turn, will pump faster to try and carry on pushing the blood around the body. Blood that has an unhealthy level of fat in its make-up will leave fatty deposits along the route. These will slowly build up and gradually reduce the blood-carrying capacity of the system. This condition is often referred to as 'furring' of the arteries or 'atherosclerosis'. By exercising regularly and monitoring our intake of fatty foods we can keep our blood-fat levels at a healthy status.

Blood Pressure

Very simply, this is the pressure exerted by the blood against the blood vessels to force the blood around the body. The average blood pressure for a healthy young adult is approximately 120/80. A blood pressure reading consistently below 140/90 is regarded as normal. A reading higher than this should be referred for medical assessment

Blood pressure levels vary throughout the day according to our lifestyle habits (activity levels, smoking, caffeine intake etc). Regular blood pressure readings can give an indication of the health of the heart and circulatory system, and certain aspects of ill health can be very quickly gauged. Very low blood pressure can lead to feelings of dizziness or vagueness, and very high blood pressure can be a sign of heart or blood circulation disease. But stress and emotional upset can also disturb your blood pressure. If in doubt, always check with your GP before planning any new exercise or activity.

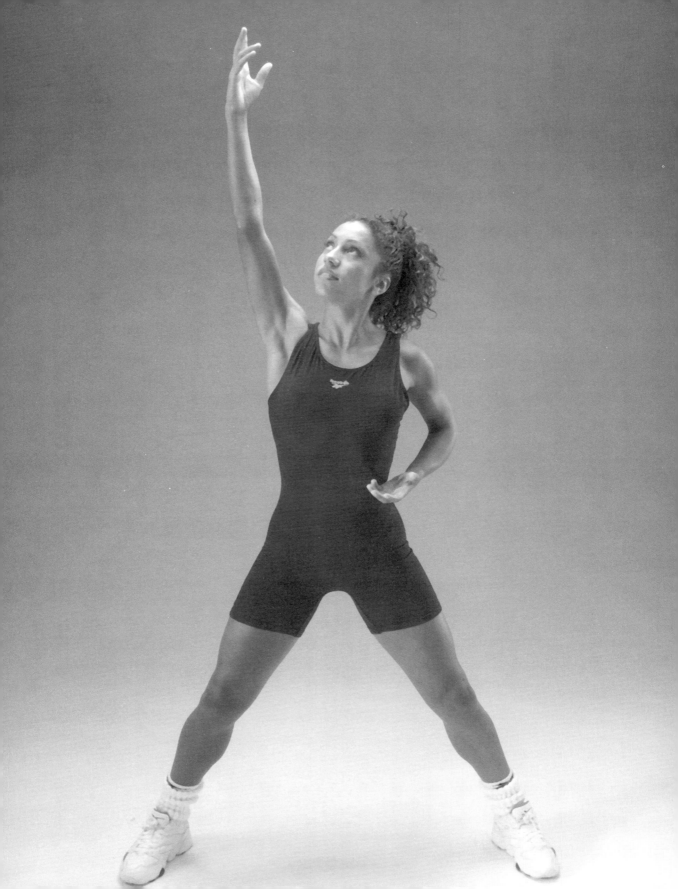

Part Two

Fitness Training Principles

Quantity and Quality

Merely going to the occasional fitness class or taking a stroll in the fresh air will get you out of the house but will not necessarily improve your fitness level. To be beneficial, aerobic exercise must meet certain criteria. It must be *frequent*, at least *three* times a week. It must last a set amount of time, at least *15 to 20 minutes*, and it must be *hard enough* – it should make you *slightly breathless* for the full 15 to 20 minutes.

The latest guidelines published by the American College of Sports Medicine suggest that to improve cardiovascular fitness you should aim to accumulate 30 minutes per day of moderate activity on most (five or six) days of the week. So, for instance, a brisk half-hour walk every weekday could help improve your aerobic fitness.

The benefits of exercising regularly can be 'lost' or reversed if, for example, you stop exercising completely or don't exercise enough. While occasional exercise may have some social or relaxation benefits, it will have very little noticeable effect in improving your aerobic fitness level. Frequency is the key word and 'little and often' is now becoming a popular prescription for the inactive population.

However, we all need to start somewhere, and it's perfectly acceptable to use exercise for social or relaxation reasons. But it's important to have a clear understanding of the true benefits of the different levels of exercise for people with different levels of fitness.

For example, a half-mile walk at a slow, strolling pace would, for most healthy people, only be 'very relaxing' and merely increase the amount of oxygen to the brain as a result of being out in the open air. But for an elderly person this could be quite a strenuous activity and form a valuable part of their weekly exercise programme, offering many health improvements. This is why it's important to be honest with yourself about your existing level of activity and to have a clear understanding of the amount and type of exercise you need to do to gain fitness benefits.

Always adapt exercise to suit your level of ability and aim to take every opportunity to incorporate activity into your daily routine. Use the stairs instead of taking the lift. Walk briskly instead of taking the bus or the car. This way, you will soon build up the ability to cope with a regular and moderate exercise programme five or six days a week.

Types of Exercise

The type of exercise you choose can be just as important to your overall success factor as the frequency, duration and intensity. Different types of exercise incorporate the different fitness components we looked at earlier and therefore provide different benefits. Unless you have a specific area that you want to work on, such as improving your strength, then you should aim for at least three sessions a week of aerobic exercise, supplemented by some strength, flexibility and relaxation work.

Selecting a form of exercise to suit your needs is not always easy. Not only are there many types of exercise but the names of the programmes and classes offered can also vary from club to club. Here is a brief overview of the different types of exercise and classes.

Aerobic Exercise

'Aerobic' is a word coined from a scientific term that means 'with oxygen' and is used to describe exercise that makes the body demand a greater amount of oxygen. It involves long periods of continuous exercise using the major muscle groups.

Aerobic exercise forms the stamina-building section of a training programme. It improves cardiovascular (aerobic) fitness, which helps prevent coronary heart disease, circulatory and respiratory problems, and is a useful tool for weight control. The best rule of thumb to determine if you are working hard enough 'aerobically' is to note for how long you are out of breath. For an aerobic workout to be effective it will have to make you slightly breathless for at least 15 to 20 minutes without stopping. If you find yourself gasping for breath, then you are working too hard. On the other hand, if you are not breathing harder during the exercise than you normally would at rest, then you are not working hard enough to train your cardiovascular system.

Beware, some aerobics classes can make you very hot and sweaty, particularly if they include lots of arm movements or complicated choreography. In this situation you might well be raising your heart rate but not become slightly breathy, so there is no guarantee that you would be getting an effective aerobic workout (although you might be getting some muscular strength and endurance training).

Examples of typical aerobic exercise include at least 15 to 20 minutes of running, jogging, fitness walking (e.g. Walk Reebok), slide training (e.g. Slide Reebok), step training (e.g. Step Reebok), aerobics classes and some of the more vigorous types of dance classes.

Anaerobic Exercise

Anaerobic means 'without oxygen', as usually happens when you run as hard as you can until you are gasping for breath. This type of exercise is therefore short and sharp. It contributes to cardiovascular fitness and is frequently used by athletes to increase their capacity for speed and power sports and enhance their performance. However, instructors or personal trainers may sometimes use this type of exercise with more advanced exercisers in the form of what we call interval training (see page 23).

Examples of typical anaerobic exercise include short, fast sprints as in running, cycling or swimming; fast ball games such as squash.

Calisthenics

This is the name given to a selection of rhythmical and repetitive movements using the weight of the body or arms or legs as resistance, as in the old-fashioned physical training class. It could also be applied to keep fit, aerobics or step classes. Calisthenics offers all-round fitness benefits and can be used to improve agility, mobility, coordination, muscle tone and cardiovascular fitness.

Flexibility Exercise

This kind of work focuses on the development of mobility in the joints and the loosening up of tight muscles. It also improves posture and range of movement. There are specific training methods to get the best from flexibility exercises with the least possible risk of injury. It is always a good idea to go to a qualified fitness instructor before embarking on your own programme of stretching and limbering.

Examples of flexibility and mobility classes include yoga, Medau, keep fit, stretch and tone. Most aerobics, step and slide classes also incorporate a period of stretching and mobilizing.

Resistance Exercise

This refers to all types of muscular strength and endurance training using resistance, usually in the form of weights, bands or tubing but sometimes using one's own body weight. Resistance exercise improves posture as well as increasing muscle tone and mass, which speeds up the calorie-burning process.

Examples of typical resistance exercise include weight-training, body-building, weight-lifting, using weight machines in a gym or health club, push-ups and abdominal strength exercises. Names given to resistance exercise classes may include bodysculpt, sculpt and tone, body conditioning and body toning.

Types of Training

Each aspect of fitness can be improved by specific methods of training, and being aware of these can help you achieve your fitness or weight-loss goals more easily.

Specificity Training

Specificity training simply means using a specific aspect of fitness training to achieve a specific goal. For instance, if you want to improve your aerobic fitness, then you need to do aerobic exercise, or if you want to improve your strength, then you need to do strength training. Because the body will adapt to whatever task or challenge you ask it to do, once it becomes accustomed to doing that particular activity on a regular basis, it becomes proficient at it.

However, although three sessions a week of weight-lifting will improve your muscular strength and endurance, it won't make great inroads into your cardiovascular endurance. There is no direct crossover. If you want to train for a specific sport or event, then you need to practise and train in that sport, so if you want to improve your tennis backhand, you need to practise your backhand technique. If you want to train to run a marathon, you need to practise and build up distance-running. However, if you want to improve your aerobic fitness so that you don't get so out of breath on the tennis court then you can cross train.

Cross Training

Cross training – sometimes called complementary training – is where you train a specific fitness component to help improve another activity. For example, if you want to improve the strength in your legs to help you cycle faster, you may choose to use the leg weight machines in a gym in addition to your cycling practice.

Interval Training

Sometimes called multiple-peak training, this is where the exercise is split into high-intensity sessions and rest sessions. For example, interval running might involve running as hard as you can for one minute and then walking to recover for three minutes. In the case of a resistance programme it might involve lifting weights for 30 seconds, then resting for 15 seconds. Interval training can be used to add variety to an exercise programme, as a tool for enhancing performance, or it can be planned to focus on a specific goal.

Circuit Training

This is used for the all-round development of each fitness component. A circuit can be any combination of equipment or free-standing exercises arranged around circuits or stations and set up in such a way that participants can move from one station to the next without interrupting the intensity level of the exercise. Circuits can be set up to allow the individual to alternate between upper body and lower body work, to balance aerobic work with resistance work, or simply to add variety to your workout as in some step circuits.

How to Progress

Everybody has a fitness training threshold – the level to which an individual can exercise and still feel comfortable. However, in order to gain benefits, you have to challenge this threshold so that you reach the slightly uncomfortable stage. This is what is called the overload principle. For example, to increase muscle strength, the muscles need to do more work than they are accustomed to doing. Since the body can very easily re-acclimatize to the new level of workload, the muscles soon begin to tone up. Then, after a period of consolidation and as soon as you begin to get 'comfortable' with this new level of workload, you need to increase the challenge again in order for the progress to continue.

The same principle applies to each fitness component, be it flexibility, cardiovascular endurance or muscular strength and endurance.

Increasing the Frequency, Duration and Intensity

To improve your fitness level you need to keep increasing the challenges. But it need not just be the intensity level (how hard the exercise is) that is increased. Benefits can also be gained from exercising more frequently or for longer periods of time. It's always advisable to increase only *one* element at a time, the frequency, duration or intensity. This way, you will achieve optimal fitness gains with the minimum risk of injury.

The accepted recommendation for maintaining fitness is to exercise three to five times a week for at least 15 to 20 minutes, to a level that keeps you slightly breathless. Increasing the frequency will give recognizable improvements quite quickly, but it is advisable to allow at least one day a week to rest.

Increasing the duration of the workout according to your ability will also show rapid improvements if you are able to maintain sufficient intensity for the full length of the workout. How hard your workout needs to be will depend on your current level of fitness.

Overtraining

Working too hard can lead to injuries. Technique, posture and reactions are poor in a tired body, and mishaps such as twisted knees and ankles are more likely to occur. In addition, because the mind and body are exhausted, the immune system is weakened, leaving the body with fewer defences against mild bugs, colds and flu. Fatigued bodies also take longer to recover from injury or illness.

Symptoms of overtraining can include dizziness, severe breathlessness, nausea, an extremely high heart rate, extreme fatigue, and tightness in the chest. (If you experience any of these symptoms you are advised to consult your doctor.)

Rest

Rest is one of the undersold factors of fitness training. For someone who is exercising regularly, it is more beneficial to exercise every other day, thus allowing time for the muscles and mind to recuperate, than it is to exercise every day. And very often your performance is enhanced after a day's rest. Top athletes always ensure their programme allows for sufficient recuperation time.

Monitoring the Intensity of Your Workout

Three of the most practical methods of measuring the intensity of your workout are perceived exertion, the talk test, and heart-rate monitoring.

Perceived Exertion

Here, the aim is to assess how hard you are working by how hard the workout feels and rate yourself according to the perceived exertion chart below. Obviously, the more experienced you become at exercising, the more accurately you are able to judge how hard you are working out. For most people, this is a reasonably accurate method of assessment and is easy to monitor in any given situation. However, it is only suitable for adults, as a child's self-perception tends to be less accurate.

The Talk Test

This self-assessment test is frequently used by professional instructors who want to keep an eagle eye on participants. The aim is to be able to hold a somewhat breathy conversation while exercising. If you are unable to talk, you need to lighten the workload a little. On the other hand, if you can recite the whole of last night's episode of your favourite soap, then you are not pushing yourself hard enough!

Heart-rate Monitoring

Monitoring your heart rate can give a good indication of the intensity of your workout, providing the exercise does not involve lifting weights, excessive arm movements or complicated choreography. These will all increase the heart rate but not necessarily increase your oxygen consumption (aerobic work) by the same rate. To monitor your heart rate there are three main factors with which you need to be familiar.

*Rate of Perceived Exertion (RPE)	
Rating	How does the exercise feel?
0	Nothing at all
0.5	Very, very weak
1	Very weak
2	Weak
3	Moderate
4	Somewhat strong
5	Strong
6	
7	Very strong
8	
9	
10	Very, very strong

* Modified Borg scale

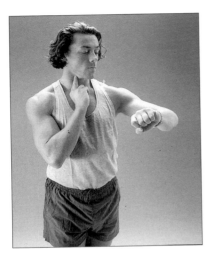

Carotid pulse.

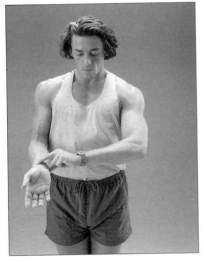

Radial pulse.

1 *Your resting heart rate (RHR)* is an indication of your lowest level of heart-beats, and is determined by taking your pulse in the morning as soon as you wake up. Take this for 60 seconds at either the throat (carotid pulse) or on the wrist (radial pulse) to determine your heart rate per minute. As you become fitter, the number of beats will decrease.

2 *Your training heart rate zone* is the range within which your heart needs to work for a consistent period of time to improve your cardiovascular fitness. To determine your training heart rate, you need to take your pulse during exercise, or as near as possible to the key part of the aerobic activity. As soon as you slow down the exercise your heart rate will drop, so you only need to take your pulse for ten seconds. Compare it to the chart on page 27, or multiply the result by six to get your heart rate over one minute.

3 *Your recovery heart rate* is how long it takes your heart rate to return to normal, which is a good indicator of your fitness level. To establish this, take your pulse at the end of the exercise cool-down. The greater your level of cardiovascular fitness, the quicker your heart rate and breathing rate will return to normal (usually one to two minutes after you have stopped exercising).

Your recovery heart rate must be taken at the same number of minutes after the aerobic section in order to be accurately used as a guide for improved fitness. Continue to cool down until your recovery heart rate is less than 100 beats per minute.

The most accurate method of monitoring your heart rate is to wear a heart-rate monitor as you exercise. The monitor straps around your chest and is attached to a wrist watch which registers your heart rate.

The aim is to gauge what your heart rate is doing at certain stages of exercise in order to try and maintain your *training heart rate zone*. It also enables you to monitor your *recovery heart rate*.

It can be quite motivating to see exactly how your heart rate changes as you perform different exercises – you'll be surprised how easy it is to increase it by working harder.

Less accurate, but equally useful, is simply to take your pulse at certain points during the workout, although some people find it hard to count the beats accurately especially if there is loud music blaring away in the background.

Finding Your Training Heart Rate Zone

Your training heart rate, which is worked out as a percentage of what we call your *maximal heart rate reserve (MHRR)*, ensures that you can maintain the exercise for a while at a workable level of intensity. The recommended percentages for your maximal heart rate reserve fall between 50 and 85. All newcomers to exercise should start at the lower end of their training heart rate zone and build up gradually as their aerobic fitness improves.

To work out your own training heart rate zone, use the following simple formula:

220 minus your age, minus your resting heart rate (RHR).
Multiply by your training percentage, add on your resting heart rate (RHR) and
divide by six.
(Dividing by six gives you a ten-second heart rate count.)

Let's calculate the training heart rate zone for a 40-year-old with a resting heart rate of 60 beats per minute (bpm) and a 50 per cent maximal heart rate reserve to establish the range or training zone within which this individual will need to work to obtain benefits without working too hard:

$$220 - 40 = 180 - 60 = 120 \times 0.5 \ (50\%) = 60 + 60 = 120 \div 6 = 20$$

For the same individual, an 85 per cent maximal heart rate reserve would produce the following result:

$$220 - 40 = 180 - 60 = 120 \times 0.85 \ (85\%) = 120 + 60 = 162 \div 6 = 27$$

Therefore this person's training heart rate zone is between 20 and 27 for a ten-second pulse rate count.

The following table provides an easy reference for participants wishing to determine a training heart rate zone between 50 and 85 per cent of MHRR.

Training Heart Rate Zone

Age	Resting Heart Rate							
	50	55	60	65	70	75	80	85
15	21–30	22–30	22–31	23–31	23–31	23–31	24–31	24–31
20	21–30	21–30	22–30	22–30	23–30	23–30	23–30	24–30
25	20–29	21–29	21–29	22–29	22–29	23–30	23–30	23–30
30	20–28	20–28	21–28	21–29	22–29	22–29	23–29	23–29
35	20–28	20–28	20–28	21–28	21–28	22–28	22–28	23–28
40	19–27	20–27	20–27	20–27	21–27	21–27	22–28	22–28
45	19–26	19–26	20–26	20–26	20–26	21–27	21–27	22–27
50	18–25	19–25	19–26	20–26	20–26	20–26	21–26	21–26
55	18–25	18–25	19–25	19–25	20–25	20–25	20–25	21–25
60	18–24	18–24	18–24	19–24	19–24	20–25	20–25	20–25
65	17–23	18–23	18–23	18–24	19–24	19–24	20–24	20–24
70	17–23	17–23	18–23	18–23	18–23	19–23	19–23	20–23
75	16–22	17–22	17–22	18–22	18–22	18–22	19–23	19–23
80	16–21	16–21	17–21	17–21	18–22	18–22	18–22	19–22

To use the above chart, locate the row that is closest to your age and find the column that corresponds to your resting heart rate. Where the row and column intersect, you will find your ten-second training heart rate zone. When you take your pulse for ten seconds during the 'working' phase of your exercise session your heart rate should fall between the figures you have found on this chart. If it falls higher, you may need to slow down a little. If it falls below this zone, you may need to try harder.

Remember, taking your pulse is only an approximate guideline to the intensity at which you are working. It is important always to follow the advice of your fitness instructor or GP.

How Active Are You?

'We tend to *overestimate* the amount of exercise we do, just as we *underestimate* the amount of food we eat! The latest thinking is that any activity is better than none – as long as it's frequent. It's better to do a little moderate activity every day, or on most days of the week, than to do nothing at all.

Activity and Health

An active lifestyle is increasingly linked to health benefits. The risks to health come from being completely sedentary or mistaking a *busy* lifestyle for an *active* one. So many of us spend our lives rushing from pillar to post (usually in a car) that we assume we have an active lifestyle. The truth is that some of that rushing about can do us more harm than good. Equally, although some of the tasks we undertake in our working lives may be physically demanding, they are not necessarily beneficial to our health and wellbeing. For example, shop assistants who spend most of the day on their feet may arrive home exhausted, feeling they have had a day full of physical activity. In fact, most likely they were placing undue stress on a body that perhaps could not cope with it.

Standing or sitting all day with little moving about means that the muscles are kept in one position for long periods of time, preventing good blood flow and thus limiting the supply of oxygen to the muscles and brain (this is why we get sleepy). In addition, holding the body in bad posture on a regular basis (many of us slouch when sitting at a desk or standing for long periods) puts strain on the back and shoulder muscles. Imagine, then, if this happens every day, the body is put at a great disadvantage and its function begins to become impaired. We start to develop all kinds of symptoms – anything from a lessened defence against the common cold, to circulation problems.

Increasing your activity level is easier than you may think, but first you need to look at your existing activity level.

Why do so few people exercise?

(Pick the excuse most familiar to you.)

+ Not enough time.
+ No one to look after the children.
+ No gym near me.

Factfile

+ **One out of every six people lead sedentary lifestyles (i.e. do not undertake any moderate or vigorous physical activity for more than 20 minutes in any four-week period).**

+ **Most people do less physical activity than necessary in order to maintain basic health and fitness levels.**

+ **Less than 85 per cent of the population do any physical activity as part of their daily workload.**

+ **Only four out of ten people participate in any regular physical activity.**

+ **We do less and less activity the older we become.**

✦ I'm too fat/thin.
✦ I'm not very coordinated.
✦ I hated PE at school.
✦ I can't afford the gear.
✦ I'm too tired/young/old/self-conscious.
✦ It's all too trendy.
✦ I don't want big muscles.

All of the above are perfectly genuine reasons for not exercising (many of us have used one or more of these at some time), so don't feel bad if you can relate to more than one of them. The good news is that we can overcome all of them – admittedly, some more easily than others – but let's start by just aiming to use them less frequently.

Assess Your Own Activity Level

In order to adopt a more active lifestyle it is important to establish how active you are at the moment. Use the following test to assess your current level and to help you determine your start point for your new level of activity.

Section One: How Active Are You?

Rate yourself according to the guidelines on page 30. Be as honest as you can – you are the only one who will miss out if you're not.

You can include both your social and work activities. For example, does your daily job involve walking? Do you dance regularly, either at an evening class or socially? How long do you do any of these things for? And how do you feel when you do each one of them?

Types of activities that count

✦ Walking to work/to the shops.
✦ Walking the dog.
✦ Walking for pleasure or transport.
✦ Walking as part of your job.
✦ Hill walking/rambling.
✦ Sweeping, mowing, any physical cleaning or decorating.
✦ Physical or manual labour such as gardening, building, farm labouring
   (but not sitting or driving machinery).
✦ Playing a sport.
✦ Exercise classes.
✦ Dance classes or social dancing (providing you do it regularly).
✦ Cycling for pleasure or transport.
✦ Swimming.

'A sedentary lifestyle is as much of a risk factor for disease as high blood pressure, obesity and smoking.'

Dr Blair, epidemiologist for the Cooper Institute for Aerobics Research, USA.

Frequency

Q	How often are you active?	Rating
	Daily or almost daily	5
	Three to five times per week	4
	One to two times per week	3
	Less than four times per month	2
	Less than once a month	1

Duration

Q	For how long does each period of activity last?	
	More than 30 minutes	4
	20 to 30 minutes	3
	10 to 20 minutes	2
	Under 10 minutes	1

Intensity

Q	How do you feel while you are being active?	
	Does your regular activity give you any of the following sensations? If you do a variety of activities, list the most frequent sensation.	
	Sustained heavy breathing and sweating	5
	Intermittent heavy breathing and sweating	4
	Moderately heavy breathing and sweating	3
	Moderate breathing, no sweating	2
	Light work, no change to breathing, no sweating	1

Calculate your score by multiplying your ratings for each aspect of the activity (frequency x duration x intensity = score). For example if you scored 3 for frequency, 3 for duration and 2 for intensity, your score would look like this: 3 x 3 x 2 = 18.

Example Sue is a shop assistant. She lives a half a mile away from her work and walks to work every day, which takes about 15 minutes. Sue then spends all day on her feet, but it's a small shop so she doesn't move very much, and she gets the bus home. She swims on Wednesday nights for 20 minutes and goes dancing every Saturday night without fail. The swimming and walking makes her slightly breathless but not sweaty. The dancing on the weekend is both hot and sweaty but doesn't make her breathless and she only does it for a few minutes at a time. Sue's score looks like this:

		Rating
Frequency	Does something nearly every day	5
Intensity	Moderate breathing, no sweating	2
Duration	Each activity takes between 10 and 20 minutes	2

Score: 5 x 2 x 2 = 20

Despite all the activity Sue undertakes in a week she still falls into the *inactive* category when we calculate her score.

Now check your scores to find your activity level.

Score	Activity Level	Start Point
Under 20	Sedentary	Level 1/Absolute Beginners
20–40	Inactive	Level 2/Beginners
40–60	Acceptable	Level 3/Intermediate
60–80	Active	Level 4/Intermediate Plus
100+	Very Active	Level 5/Advanced

You can also use this test to check your progress. Repeat it after six weeks on your new healthy lifestyle to see how much more activity you are doing, and what your new score is.

Section Two:
What Kind of Activity is Right for You?

Now that you know your activity level and start point you need to identify the right kind and amount of exercise appropriate to you. Most fitness instructors or clubs will rate their classes using terms similar to those above. But always check with the instructor first to make sure the level is right for you as this can vary from club to club. Here is a further guide to the intensity of sporting and everyday activities based on a minimum duration of 15 to 20 minutes.

*Suitable for Levels 1–2 (1 to 3 times a week)
Light Activities: Long walks of two miles or more at a comfortable pace (3 mph); light decorating; table tennis; golf; ballroom or recreational dancing; light gardening; badminton; recreational swimming.

*Suitable for Levels 2–4 (3 to 4 times a week)
Moderate Activities: Long walks of two miles or more at a brisk or fast pace; football; swimming (several lengths at a time); tennis; movement classes; low-impact aerobics and recreational dancing to intermediate level or for at least an hour (it should also make you out of breath and sweaty); heavy gardening (e.g. digging); heavy housework (e.g. spring cleaning).

*Suitable for Levels 4–5 (3 to 6 times a week)
Vigorous Activities: Hill walking at a brisk pace; squash; running (including that involved in sports); football; tennis; aerobics; step training; slide training; competitive dancing; cycling. (All these activities should make you out of breath and sweaty.)

* Based on the classification of activity from the Allied Dunbar National Fitness Survey, England, 1992.

Health Status

Once you have determined your activity level, you need to assess your health status before starting an exercise programme. For most people, taking up exercise will bring added pleasure and improvements to their health and social life. Some may need to seek the advice of their GP before starting a new activity, particularly those people who have not been active for some time, or who are pregnant, smoke, take certain prescribed drugs, have certain ailments or disorders or who are over 40.

It is important, therefore, that you complete the following questionnaire before you consider joining a class or increasing your exercise level.

Health History Evaluation

1   Do you have a history of any of the following conditions?

Heart problem	Yes ☐	No ☐
High blood pressure	Yes ☐	No ☐
High cholesterol	Yes ☐	No ☐
Respiratory problems	Yes ☐	No ☐
Diabetes	Yes ☐	No ☐
Surgery within the last three months	Yes ☐	No ☐
Major illnesses or hospitalization in the last three months	Yes ☐	No ☐
Major muscle, joint or back disorder	Yes ☐	No ☐
Any other physical problem needing special attention	Yes ☐	No ☐

2   Are you over 40 years of age?   Yes ☐   No ☐

3   Are you significantly overweight?   Yes ☐   No ☐

4   Are you pregnant?   Yes ☐   No ☐

5   Are you taking any medication?   Yes ☐   No ☐

If you answered 'yes' to any of the above questions it is essential you check with your GP before embarking on any form of exercise.

Planning Your Fitness Menu

Once you have assessed your activity level, and you've got the all-clear or the relevant advice from your GP, the next stage is to plan your programme for a healthier, fitter lifestyle.

Motivation

Lack of motivation and adherence (not dropping out of your exercise programme) are two of the biggest problems recognized by fitness professionals worldwide. But there are steps you can take to give yourself the best chance of enjoying your exercise programme so that you want to continue.

Goal Setting

It's very important to ask yourself 'why am I doing this?' (You will probably ask yourself this question on many occasions!) But knowing what you want to achieve and what are your personal goals is essential if you are to plan a successful programme of activity that will keep you motivated and give you the desired results.

Personality plays an important part. If you are the sort of person that enjoys being in a group, then solitary running or working out at home is not going to make you happy or keep you exercising. So be clear about your preferences and what you want from your exercise programme.

Once you have identified your reasons for embarking on your new exercise campaign you can then set some more specific goals.

Personal Goals

I want to lose weight.

I want to put on some weight.

I want to get fitter.

I want to be able to climb the stairs to my office without getting out of breath.

I want to improve my game of squash/tennis/football.

I want to have more energy.

I want to get away from the children/family/work.

I want a girls'/boys' night out.

I want to be able to tie my own shoe laces in old age.

I want to be able to stay the course on our next hiking holiday.

I want to enter a cycling race.

I want to walk for charity.

I want to tone up my legs/buttocks/stomach.

I want to be able to wear a swimsuit this summer.

I want to quit smoking.

S.M.A.R.T.

The next step is to put together a plan of action, using the S.M.A.R.T. method, to help you achieve your goals. Keep in mind the following guidelines as you plot your campaign.

S is for Specific. Many people fail on exercise programmes because their goals are not specific enough. Define your goals clearly so you have a firm idea of what you want to achieve. Write them down on a piece of paper, listing them in order of priority, for example:

1. Lose ten pounds.
2. Walk a ten kilometre race.
3. Improve flexibility in hips.
4. Improve tennis backhand.

M is for Measurable. There is nothing more exciting than being able to see your progress, and this is certain to keep you motivated. So, be sure to make your goals measurable. There are many ways of doing this. On the first day you start out on your new healthy lifestyle measure yourself and enter your vital statistics on the chart on page 151. Next, make a note of how far or for how long you can comfortably walk or run (e.g. how long does it take you to walk a mile?) and set yourself some preliminary goals. Repeat these simple tests a few weeks later and reassess your activity level (see page 29) to see how far you have progressed.

A is for Action. Don't just think about it – do it! Plan each step you need to take to get yourself to the gym or exercise class. Draw up an action plan, for example:

1. Call health club to book a tour of the club.
2. Call friend and ask him/her to come with you for support.
3. Book appointment with GP for a full check-up. (Ensure blood pressure is measured.)
4. Dig out sports shoes from the loft.
5. Plan your chosen programme of exercise (establish what type, and how often, for how long and how hard you should work out).

Remember to tick each one off as you work your way through the list.

R is for Realistic. Don't aim too high or you will only feel dejected if you don't achieve what you set out to do. Split major goals into small 'bite-size' pieces. For example, if you feel you'll never shift that extra weight you've gained over the last two years, don't aim to lose the whole amount in one go. Instead, give yourself a target of, say, five pounds at a time. Each time you succeed in losing five pounds, give yourself a pat on the back. After all, you have achieved something worthwhile and are getting closer and closer to your long-term goal.

T is for Timed. Set yourself a time limit. Again, make sure it is realistic. Can you really shift five pounds in just one week? Unlikely – and inadvisable from a health point of view – so give yourself a month. And if it looks as though you will exceed your goal in the stated time, don't change anything – just keep going. It's far better to come in ahead of target than to increase the challenges halfway through. Without a time limit you may tend to forget your goal or let it meander on for too long. Having a time limit also allows you to measure how well you've done in a certain period of time. Special events provide good motivators, but give yourself plenty of time to work towards them. There's nothing more disappointing than having that special day loom closer, and not being able to lose that five pounds in time.

Tips to Keep You Motivated

1. Use the S.M.A.R.T. method to plan your goals.
2. Chart your progress so that you have a visible record of the changes that are taking place.
3. Ask your family and friends for support.
4. Don't try to conquer the world in a day. Instead, aim for small but important changes.
5. Be positive – you can achieve whatever you want if you set your mind to it.

> **Tip**
>
> Small changes can make a big difference. For instance, walking for an extra 15 minutes each day gives a total of nearly two hours additional exercise each week!

We all need encouragement to help us achieve our goals. Make sure those around you know how important this is to you. Adopting a positive attitude will give you a greater chance of success. So be proud of each small gain you make and steer clear of anyone who tries to put you off your goal or who belittles your achievement.

Balancing the Challenge

Now that you know what your goals are, the next stage is to select the best type of exercise programme or activity to achieve those goals – one that suits your personality and lifestyle. Different types of exercise offer different benefits, so before signing up for a session at a health club or gym it's important to look at what is available and what that particular activity is likely to help you achieve.

Some forms of sport or exercise are better than others for improving flexibility, while other activities may produce greater aerobic training benefits. Remember, the body works on a very simple learning process – the more you ask it do one specific task, the better it becomes at doing that particular task.

What to Aim For

Unless you have some specific goal in mind such as improved flexibility, weight loss or a special sporting event, most people need to aim for an all-round, balanced approach to working out – one which takes into account all the fitness components. For a balanced workout you should aim to include activities that improve your cardiovascular fitness, strength and flexibility.

If you encounter a great deal of stress in any particular week you can also add a relaxation session. Remember, the aim is to build up your activity gradually to a minimum of 30 minutes on most days of the week.

So, you may start out by exercising just two to three days a week and build up a weekly schedule that looks something like the one on the right:

Use the chart on page 154 to plot your weekly schedule and monitor your progress. Remember, whatever you choose to do, you must build up gradually. If you are a complete beginner, start off by exercising on two to three days a week, and gradually add more days. Follow the safety guidelines in the next section to ensure you get the best from your new exercise programme.

Sample Weekly Schedule	
Monday	Step class (e.g. Step Reebok®)
Tuesday	Swimming or Basic Workout (see page 51)
Wednesday	Step class
Thursday	Fitness walking (e.g. Walk Reebok)
Friday	Rest
Saturday	Slide class (e.g. Slide Reebok™)
Sunday	Family cycle or walk

Preparing to Exercise

While the test on page 29 will give you an idea of your current level of activity, a fitness assessment will measure specific components of fitness to enable you to design a personalized exercise programme.

Fitness Assessments

These analyse posture and measure cardiovascular (aerobic) fitness, flexibility, muscular strength and endurance and body composition. All can be carried out by a fitness professional at your local health club or leisure facility. On the following pages you will find a few simple tests that you can apply yourself. Remember to warm up thoroughly before attempting the aerobic fitness and strength assessments. Again, if you answered 'yes' to any of the questions in the Health History Evaluation questionnaire, you should check with your doctor before trying any of these tests.

Remember to note the results of your first assessments on the progress chart on page 152. Repeat the tests in a few weeks time and record any improvements you have made.

Tip

If you ask your local health club for a fitness assessment, ensure they talk you through the whole procedure so that you understand what is happening throughout the various tests.

Posture Analysis

Correct posture is crucial to injury prevention, not only when exercising, but also in everyday life. Good posture benefits health by allowing the internal organs to function more efficiently and the muscles to work effectively and safely. Poor posture can lead to joint strains such as in the ankle and hip and also cause severe back problems, which are particularly prevalent in the western world.

The body is designed to stand upright which allows for the most efficient performance. Unfortunately, since most of us spend a great deal of the day sitting down – either behind a desk or the wheel of a car – the postural muscles (those that specifically help us to stand up straight) become very lax. In turn, this compromises our joint action, and leaves us vulnerable to injury.

And a sedentary job or inactive lifestyle are not the only contributory factors. Poor posture may also be attributed to ongoing stress. Individuals who are continually fatigued or stressed can be easily identified by the way they carry themselves: shoulders slumped, tight neck and shoulder muscles or hamstrings.

Most postural problems are easily remedied by a little conscious practice in standing and sitting correctly, or by some specific stretching and strengthening of the postural muscles. But the first step is to identify your own posture habits.

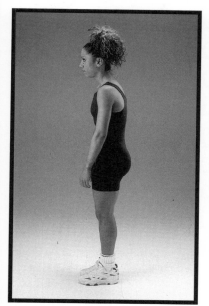

Poor posture.

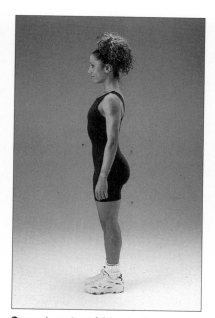

Correct posture (side view).

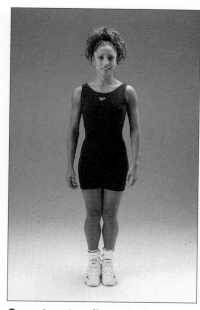

Correct posture (front view).

The Posture Test

1. Stand in front of a full-length mirror and strip down to your underwear – or, even better, take off all your clothes, if you're brave enough.

2. Stand face on to the mirror and take a good look at the way you stand. Answer the questions on the following page.

3. Turn sideways on to the mirror (this position really reveals the bad habits) and do the same.

4. Draw the imaginary lines that relate to your own posture lines.

Factfile

✦ It's a myth that only dancers and models can have good posture. Everyone can improve their posture through exercise.

✦ Good posture can make you appear taller, slimmer and more confident.

Posture Questionnaire

Face on

			Your comments
✦ Are your shoulders level?	Yes ☐	No ☐	
Left shoulder higher/lower?	Higher ☐	Lower ☐	
Right shoulder higher/lower?	Higher ☐	Lower ☐	
✦ Are your hips level?	Yes ☐	No ☐	
Left hip higher/lower?	Higher ☐	Lower ☐	
Right hip higher/lower?	Higher ☐	Lower ☐	
✦ Are your knees level?	Yes ☐	No ☐	
Left knee higher/lower?	Higher ☐	Lower ☐	
Right knee higher/lower?	Higher ☐	Lower ☐	
Kneecaps turning inward/outward?	Inward ☐	Outward ☐	
✦ Are your ankles rolling in/out?	In ☐	Out ☐	
✦ Do you have flat feet/high arches?	Flat ☐	High arches ☐	
Feet turned in/out?	In ☐	Out ☐	

Sideways on

If you are standing correctly you should be able to draw a straight line from your ear-lobe down through the centre of your shoulder, hip, knee and ankle joints. If you can't, you may have one or more of the following alignment problems.

			Your comments
✦ Does your chin jut forward?	Yes ☐	No ☐	
✦ Are your shoulders hunched forward?	Yes ☐	No ☐	
✦ Does your stomach stick out?	Yes ☐	No ☐	
✦ Is your lower back arched?	Yes ☐	No ☐	
✦ Do your knees sway back?	Yes ☐	No ☐	

If you have identified more than one alignment problem that you can't remedy instantly by just correcting your posture and standing upright, check with your doctor before embarking on any strenuous exercise programme. If you have serious postural problems, you may need to consult an osteopath, physiotherapist or Alexander technician for advice on remedial exercises.

Aerobic Fitness Assessment

The objective here is to measure your aerobic fitness so that you can determine the appropriate intensity level at which you should begin your exercise programme and thereby lessen the risk of injury. In a health club you would be asked to step or cycle for a few minutes, after which your pulse rate would be taken.

The One-mile Walking Test

1. Make sure you have completed the Health History Evaluation questionnaire. If you answered 'no' to each question, progress to 2. If you answered 'yes' to any of the questions make an appointment to see your doctor before going further.
2. You will need a good pair of walking shoes, a stop watch or a watch with a second hand, plus a pedometer to measure the distance as you walk (pedometers are available from most sports shops).
3. Do not have any caffeinated drinks for at least three hours before the test.
4. Find a smooth, level surface such as a school athletics track, a pathway in a park, shopping centre or local street where you can accurately measure a one-mile distance.
5. Warm up thoroughly by walking briskly for at least ten minutes.
6. Note the time on your watch, then begin the test by walking (not running) the one mile as quickly as possible but without straining. As you will need to keep to a constant pace for the duration of the test, be sure to set off at a pace you are confident you can maintain.
7. When you have completed the mile don't stop suddenly – keep moving and look at your watch to see how long it took and, at the same time, take your pulse for 15 seconds. Multiply the number of beats by four to determine your heart beat per minute (bpm). For example, if you counted 32 beats during the 15 seconds, your heartbeat (pulse rate) would be 128 bpm (32 x 4 = 128). Make a note of your pulse rate.
8. Make a note (in minutes and seconds) of the time it took you to walk the mile. The average time is between 10 and 20 minutes
9. Continue to walk slowly for at least five minutes to let the heart rate and blood pressure return to normal.
10. Compare your test results with the figures on the charts overleaf to determine your aerobic fitness level.

To use the one-mile walking test chart overleaf, find your age category and pulse rate. If the exact pulse rate is not shown, round it off. To the right of this is the one-mile walk times for low, medium and high fitness levels. You may need to make adjustments if your weight differs from the specified weight.

Note that for a given heart rate, the older you are, the faster you must walk to qualify for a fitness category. This is because the maximal heart rate decreases with age. Therefore, for any given heart rate, a younger person is working at a relatively lower percentage of maximum aerobic capacity than an older person.

The Cooper Institute for Aerobics Research One-mile Walking Test is used with the permission of the Cooper Institute for Aerobics Research. The fitness levels for the One-mile Walking Test are estimated from a regression equation in: Rippe JM et al, *Walking for health and fitness.* JAMA 1988; 259:2720–2724.

The One-mile Walking Test Chart

Men
Assumes weight of 175 lb

Age	Heart Rate	Low Fitness	Medium Fitness	High Fitness
20–29	110	>19:36	17:06–19:36	<17:06
	120	>19:10	16:36–19:10	<16:36
	130	>18:35	16:06–18:35	<16:06
	140	>18:06	15:36–18:06	<15:36
	150	>17:36	15:10–17:36	<15:10
	160	>17:09	14:42–17:09	<14:42
	170	>16:39	14:21–16:39	<14:12
30–39	110	>18:21	15:54–18:21	<15:54
	120	>17:52	15:24–17:52	<15:24
	130	>17:22	15:54–17:22	<14:54
	140	>16:54	14:30–16:54	<14:30
	150	>16:26	14:00–16:26	<14:00
	160	>15:58	13:30–15:58	<13:30
	170	>15:28	13:01–15:28	<13:01
40–49	110	>18:05	15:38–18:05	<15:38
	120	>17:36	15:09–17:36	<15:09
	130	>17:07	14:41–17:07	<14:41
	140	>16:38	14:12–16:38	<14:12
	150	>16:09	13:42–16:09	<13:42
	160	>15:42	13:15–15:42	<13:15
	170	>15:12	12:45–15:12	<12:45
50–59	110	>17:49	15:22–17.49	<15:22
	120	>17:20	14:53–17:20	<14:53
	130	>16:51	14:24–16:51	<14:24
	140	>16:22	13:51–16:22	<13:51
	150	>15:53	13:26–15:53	<13:26
	160	>15:26	12:59–15:26	<12:59
	170	>14:56	12:30–14:56	<12:30
60+	110	>17:55	15:33–17:55	<15:33
	120	>17:24	15:04–17:24	<15:04
	130	>16:57	14:36–16:57	<14:36
	140	>16:28	14:07–16:28	<14:07
	150	>15:59	13:39–15:59	<13:39
	160	>15:30	13:10–15:30	<13:10
	170	>15:04	12:42–15:04	<12:42

Women
*Assumes weight of 125 lb

Age	Heart Rate	Low Fitness	Medium Fitness	High Fitness
20–29	110	>20:57	19:08–20:57	<19:08
	120	>20:27	18:38–20:27	<18:38
	130	>20:00	18:12–20:00	<18:12
	140	>19:30	17:42–19:30	<17:42
	150	>19:00	17:12–19:00	<17:12
	160	>18:30	16:42–18:30	<16:42
	170	>18:00	16:12–18:00	<16:12
30–39	110	>19:46	17:52–19:46	<17:52
	120	>19:18	17:24–19:18	<17:24
	130	>18:48	16:54–18:48	<16:54
	140	>18:18	16:24–18:18	<16:24
	150	>17:48	15:54–17:48	<15:54
	160	>17:18	15:24–17:18	<15:24
	170	>16:54	14:55–16:54	<14:55
40–49	110	>19:15	17:20–19:15	<17:20
	120	>18:45	16:50–18:45	<16:50
	130	>18:18	16:24–18:18	<16:24
	140	>17:48	15:54–17:48	<15:54
	150	>17:18	15:24–17:18	<15:24
	160	>16:48	15:54–16:48	<14:54
	170	>16:18	14:25–16:18	<14:25
50–59	110	>18:40	17:04–18:40	<17:04
	120	>18:12	16:36–18:12	<16:36
	130	>17:42	16:06–17:42	<16:06
	140	>17:18	15:36–17:18	<15:36
	150	>16:48	15:06–16:48	<15:06
	160	>16:18	14:36–16:18	<14:36
	170	>15:48	14:06–15:48	<14:06
60+	110	>18:00	16:36–18:00	<16:36
	120	>17:30	16:06–17:30	<16:06
	130	>17:01	15:37–17:01	<15:37
	140	>16:31	15:09–16:31	<15:09
	150	>16:02	14:39–16:02	<14:39
	160	>15:32	14:12–15:32	<14:12
	170	>15:04	13:42–15:04	<13:42

*For every 10 lb over 175 lb, males must walk 15 seconds faster to qualify for a fitness category.

*For every 10 lb under 175 lb, males can walk 15 seconds slower to qualify for a fitness category

*For every 10 lb over 125 lb, females must walk 15 seconds faster to qualify for a fitness category.

*For every 10 lb under 125 lb, females can walk 15 seconds slower to qualify for a fitness category.

Flexibility Assessment

Assessing your own flexibility will give you a guideline as to which areas of your body need that extra bit of stretching and mobility work. Having limited flexibility can make you more prone to injury when exercising or rushing about completing your daily tasks.

Common flexibility problems include tight hamstrings, which can lead to lower back pain, especially for people who do step training, slide training or aerobics, and tight calf muscles, which can lead to ankle or Achilles problems, especially for runners and walkers.

It's important for elderly people to maintain their flexibility levels in order to be able to maintain independent lifestyles, such as being to get on and off buses, reach to brush their own hair etc.

Guidelines

1. Ask a friend or partner to help you assess your results in the tests overleaf.
2. If you are extremely overweight or suffer from back pain or joint injuries *do not* carry out these tests.
3. Follow the instructions for each test carefully and ask your friend or partner to help you estimate the range of flexibility in each of your joints. Friends or partners should assess visually only. They should not touch your limbs or interfere with your movement in any way.
4. Stretch *only* to a point of mild tension – not pain. Stretch slowly – do not bounce – and breathe normally throughout.
5. Make a note of your body areas with limited flexibility. You will need to pay special attention to these areas, since they will affect your technique in certain activities and may make you more prone to injury. Practise the relevant stretching exercises for the appropriate body part.
6. Chart your improvements in flexibility on the progress chart on page 152.

The Flexibility Tests

Test Directions	Aim	Remedy

Hip Flexors (front of hip joints)

Lying on your back, pull one knee to chest, other leg fully extended on floor.

Calf of extended leg must remain on the floor, knee must not bend.

Hip Flexor Stretch (page 88)

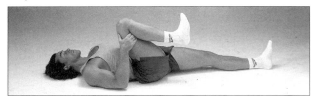

Hamstrings (back of thighs)

Lying on your back, lift one leg keeping the other leg flat on the floor without bending either knee.

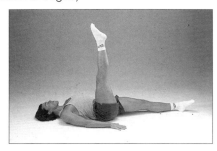

Raised leg must reach a vertical position.

Hamstring Stretch (page 62)

Quadriceps (front of thighs)

Lying on your stomach with knees together, gently pull heel towards buttocks.

Heels should comfortably touch buttocks.

Quadricep Stretch (page 63)

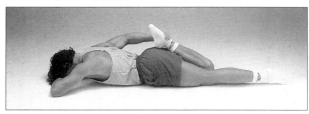

Soleus (calf)

Standing with one foot flat on a platform with the knee directly above the ankle joint, raise forefoot up off the platform, keeping the supporting knee straight but relaxed and both heels down.

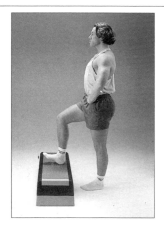

Ball of the foot should clear the platform by at least two fingers width.

Calf Stretch (page 64)

Strength Assessment

Many postural problems can be traced back to weak abdominal muscles, so, we shall concern ourselves solely with abdominal strength here. This test estimates whether you have adequate abdominal strength to maintain good posture. However, it does not distinguish between basic abdominal strength and very good abdominal strength. So even if you can hold for more than ten counts, you may still need to increase your level of abdominal work .

The Abdominal Strength Test

Lie on your back on a flat surface or the floor with knees bent and just hip-distance apart, feet flat on the floor. Your feet should not be held down by anyone or anything. Place your hands behind your head, elbows out to the sides. Without pulling on your head with your hands, slowly lift your head and shoulders off the floor, keeping the lower back in contact with the floor. Hold for 10 slow counts while breathing normally, then slowly lower the head and shoulders to the floor.

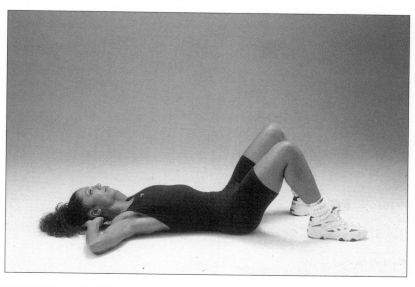

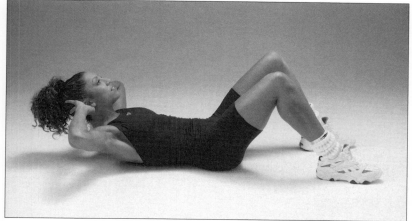

Levels of Abdominal Strength

Unable to lift head: *very poor*

Unable to lift head and shoulders: *poor*

Able to lift and hold head and shoulders for 10 counts: *adequate*

Able to lift and hold for more than 10 counts: *good*

Injury Prevention

When exercising we are placing the body under stress, so the least we can do is abide by a few well-researched guidelines to help limit the possibilities of injury.

The Safe Exercise Code

✦ Always wear the appropriate shoes and clothing.

✦ Wear extra layers of clothing in the cold and peel them off as you warm up.

✦ Always warm up thoroughly.

✦ Practise good technique and good posture.

✦ Don't attempt to do too much too soon.

✦ Progress gradually.

✦ If it hurts, don't do it.

✦ Always cool down and stretch out after exercise.

✦ When using equipment always follow the appropriate guidelines.

✦ If exercising alone out of doors make sure you leave details of where you are going and how long you intend to be.

✦ Do not exercise if feeling unwell or suffering from colds or flu.

✦ Do not exercise on existing injuries. Allow sufficient recovery time, otherwise the injury will not heal and is likely to get worse.

✦ Seek proper medical advice for all joint injuries.

✦ The R.I.C.E. method (see below) should be applied to all sudden strains and sprains.

✦ If in any doubt check with your GP.

R.I.C.E.

This is the method used by doctors and athletics coaches for immediate treatment of muscle and joint injuries. R.I.C.E. stands for Rest, Ice, Compression and Elevation. So, when an injury occurs, the action needs to be stopped and the body part rested. Ice is then applied to the injury, but never directly to the skin (cloth or fabric is placed between to form a layer) and icing is limited to ten to fifteen minutes at a time). The body part is then strapped up and elevated to help reduce the blood flow.

Warming Up and Cooling Down

Joints and muscles function best when they are healthy and warm. This is why warming up is such a crucial injury prevention tool in any workout. Serious athletes will not squander their warm-up time, since they know they are more likely to achieve a top performance with a lower risk of injury if they warm up thoroughly before putting their bodies under pressure.

The Warming Effect

An effective warm-up should

✦ increase the blood flow to the muscles

✦ increase muscle elasticity

✦ speed up the nerve message system from the brain to the limbs

✦ lubricate the joints

✦ gently raise the heart rate

✦ increase mental alertness

✦ increase the core body temperature.

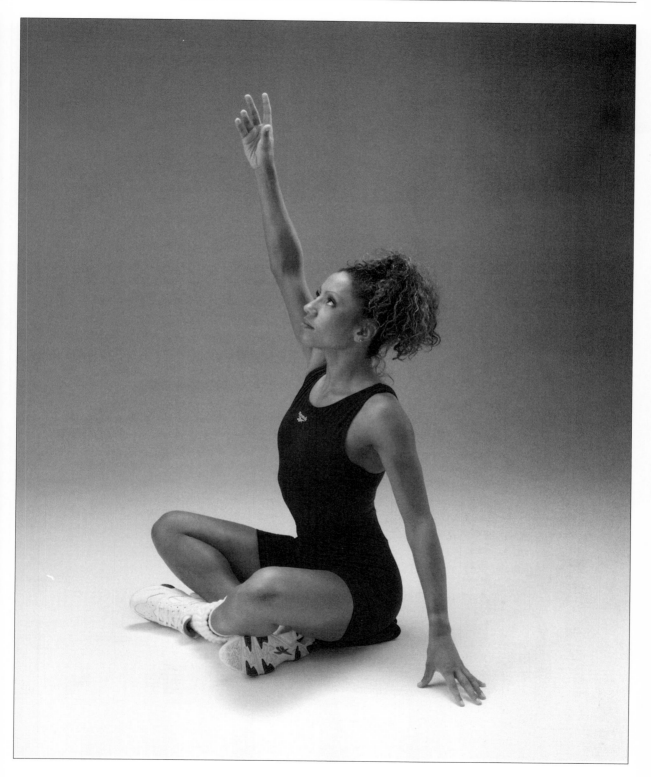

How to Warm Up

Each of the workouts included in this book has its own warm-up guidelines. A good warm-up should prepare you for the activity to follow. If devising your own warm-up, make sure you include the following elements:

1. Use light jogging or walking to raise the body temperature and breathing rate (2–3 minutes).
2. When you feel warmer, stretch out the muscles you are going to be using. See pages 62–64 for stretches (5 minutes).
3. Rehearse the activity that is to follow by gently practising the moves you will be doing and mobilizing the joints and limbs involved (1–2 minutes).

Cooling Down and Stretching

To cool down after vigorous exercise, continue to perform the activity at a lesser intensity and then stretch out the parts of the body that have done the most work. Cooling down and stretching in this way will help dissipate the build-up of waste products in the muscles and help prevent muscle soreness.

Immediately after your exercise session, while the body is still really warm, is also a good time to work on improving flexibility. Not only does this relax the body, but it also stretches the muscles and mobilizes the joints at a time when they are most receptive.

D.O.M.S.

This stands for Delayed Onset Muscle Soreness, which occurs as a result of participating in a new exercise or doing too much too soon before your muscles are capable of handling the extra work. The soreness is 'delayed' because it usually occurs most severely 24 to 48 hours after the exercise has taken place.

Gentle stretching and 'active rest' (keep active but to a lesser intensity) are usually the best cures. In other words, don't over-nurse the soreness, and don't do the activity that brought it on in the first place. The soreness should disappear within a couple of days.

Technique

Equally important when exercising, is to pay attention to your own movement technique, which means keeping the body in its correct alignment.

The correct technique for each programme in this book is detailed in the appropriate workout section. Essentially, it means that joints should always be in line with each other, as detailed in the posture test (see page 37), so that they move only in the direction in which they are designed to move.

Good technique and posture will protect the joints and minimize injury. Therefore, be sure always to follow the correct guidelines for an exercise programme and listen carefully to any instructions given in an exercise class.

Footwear for Injury Prevention

Selecting the correct footwear is important for injury prevention. Depending on the activity you are undertaking, the wrong or inadequate footwear can be as harmful as not wearing any at all. On the other hand, walking barefoot or stretching your feet and ankles without the restriction of shoes will enhance the development of strength and flexibility in your feet.

All the joints in the body, but especially the feet and ankles, are designed to withstand a certain amount of shock. The muscles and connective tissue act as natural shock absorbers and need to be kept in shape by regular barefoot work such as walking, as well as stretching and flexing the feet both when standing and sitting. But, after a certain level of impact, the feet need extra help in the shape of a well-designed pair of shoes. Here are some guidelines for selecting shoes.

✦ Choose the correct shoes for the activity you undertake most frequently. Good-quality shoes are specially designed to help take some of the stress out of that particular activity by offering cushioning and support in the appropriate places.

✦ Generally, for a heel-strike activity such as running or walking, the shoe will have more cushioning in the heel. For a forefoot-strike activity such as low- or high-impact aerobics the shoe will often have more cushioning in the ball of the foot. For a general activity choose a shoe that is well cushioned in both the heel and forefoot.

✦ Shoes for aerobic-type exercise need to be lightweight yet strong enough to support the foot as it goes through the mechanical action involved in that activity. A shoe should not interfere with the natural movement of the foot.

✦ The outsole should have an appropriate degree of traction for the surface on which the shoes will be used for both indoor and outdoor work.

✦ A good shoe for any activity will have a solid heel cup. This is essential to ensure a good fit and to ensure that the shoe moves with the foot at all times.

✦ Lacing is an important part of the support system and works to hold the whole upper portion of the shoe in the correct shape around the foot as it moves.

✦ Side panels and straps are there for a reason, usually to offer extra support for sideways twists and turns in certain sports and exercises.

✦ Breathing panels are essential for activities where participants sweat a great deal. The shoes should be ventilated to enable the feet to 'breathe'.

✦ High- or low-cut ankle collars are a question of personal preference except in sports which involve a lot of jumping, twisting and turning, such as basketball. A shoe with a high collar will offer more support to the ankle joint, but since this can also inhibit ankle movement, it should not be worn for all activities.

✦ Look after your shoes. Throwing them in the washing machine (unless specifically advised by the manufacturer) will shorten the life and the support system.

✦ Don't wear shoes where the cushioning has been worn flat or the uppers have become very supple. Worn-out shoes offer less protection and can lead to an increased risk of injury.

✦ Shoes should always fit properly. Your heels should fit snugly into the heel cup and your toes should be at least a thumb's width from the end of the 'toe' of the shoes. You should be able to wiggle your toes easily, and the collars and tongues should not rub the ankle or press against the Achilles tendon (the narrow bit at the back of the ankle joint).

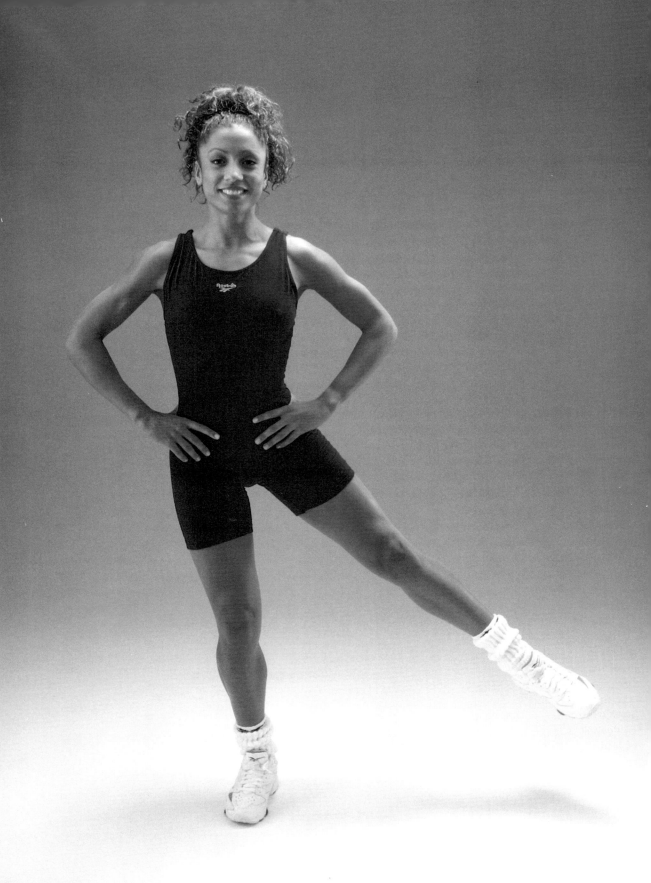

Part Three
The Training Programmes

Now that you know the benefits of exercise and how to prepare and plan your programme, this section introduces you to three popular Reebok University fitness programmes, plus a Basic Workout for the complete beginner.

Before starting any of these programmes make sure you have read through the previous chapters and completed the activity level assessment, fitness assessments and Health History Evaluation questionnaire. If you answered 'yes' to any of the questions on the health questionnaire, or if you have any other doubts or worries, please consult your GP first.

If planning to exercise at home make sure you have plenty of space and time. Move breakable objects and furniture out of the way, and take the phone off the hook so you are not interrupted. This is *your* time.

The Way It All Works

The programmes are designed so that they can work together or separately, depending on how much challenge you are ready for. Each has its own detailed guidelines on correct technique and safe exercising, plus recommendations for starting out according to your level of fitness. The aerobics section of each workout can be repeated as indicated for a more challenging workout.

How to Fit Them Together

The Basic Workout can be used as a start point for complete beginners. Alternatively, the different sections can be used in conjunction with any of the other programmes. For example:

The Novice Challenge: If you've never exercised before, follow the Basic Workout for six weeks, or until you feel confident doing it at least three times a week, before moving on to any of the other programmes.

The Getting There Challenge: Follow the Basic Workout on alternate days to the Walk Reebok, Step Reebok or Slide Reebok training programme.

The Multi Challenge: For added benefit, combine the strengthening and flexibility sections from the Basic Workout with the Walk Reebok, Step Reebok or Slide Reebok training programme.

The Extra Challenge: For extra challenge, combine the entire Basic Workout with the Walk Reebok, Step Reebok or Slide Reebok training programme.

The Super Challenge: For maximum challenge, combine the entire Basic Workout with two of the other programmes (Walk Reebok, Step Reebok or Slide Reebok).

Whichever programme you are following, always use the warm-up and stretch and the cool-down and stretch from the Basic Workout.

Weekly Planner

For each of the following programmes a suggested weekly exercise schedule is provided involving that particular programme. This is intended as a guideline only, and you should plan your weekly schedule to fit your specific needs and based on the advice in Part Two of this book. Use the weekly exercise schedule progress chart on page 154 to plot and monitor your progress.

A Word on Music

If you choose to work out to music, pay particular attention to the speed of the music you select for each section of your workout, since this will affect the intensity of the exercise. Music that is too fast will also prevent you from completing each move properly and will increase the risk of injury. Music that is too slow can make some moves laborious, or may not help you achieve your desired training level. However, if in doubt, always err on the side of caution and start off with a speed slower than that at which you intend to continue. You can always increase it when you become more confident. Recommended music speeds are included for the relevant sections of the Basic Workout, Step Reebok and Slide Reebok training programmes. Beginners should always choose a speed towards the lower end of the specified range.

Reasons to Relax

The end of the Basic Workout includes a few minutes of relaxation. This is an important aspect of good health which is often neglected. Dedicate these few minutes to yourself at the end of your workout – or even instead of your workout on those days when you just can't muster up the energy for another toe touch!

A Reminder

Remember, the warm-up and stretch is an important part of each programme. The aerobics section of each workout is designed to increase your oxygen uptake (breathing), and the cool-down and stretch will gradually bring your pulse and breathing rate down to normal and stretch out the muscles you have been working.

Follow the guidelines accurately for a great workout – and if it hurts, don't do it!

The Basic Workout

This simple workout serves as an introduction to exercising and can be used with or without music, according to preference. The warm-up and stretch and the cool-down and stretch should also be used for the same purpose in the other programmes. Learn the basic moves in the warm-up and aerobics section before you move on to the routines.

     If you choose to use the Basic Workout as your main form of exercise, your weekly schedule could look like the one below (this assumes you are at Level 2: Beginners).

Suggested Weekly Schedule

Monday	Basic Workout	30 minutes
Tuesday	Swim leisurely	30 minutes
Wednesday	Basic Workout	30 minutes
Thursday	Rest	
Friday	Walk	30 minutes
Saturday	Basic Workout	30 minutes
Sunday	Rest/leisurely stroll	60 minutes

The Basic Moves: Warm-up and Aerobic

Practise the basic moves first. When you feel comfortable with each one and can move from one to another with ease, you can then attempt the routines.
Start by standing with feet hip-distance apart, knees slightly bent, and maintain this stance throughout the moves. In the first five moves, keep the feet stationary.

Shoulder Rolls ▶

Roll both shoulders backward. Really feel them loosen up (4 counts). Repeat, rolling both shoulders forward.

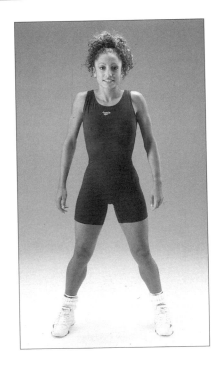
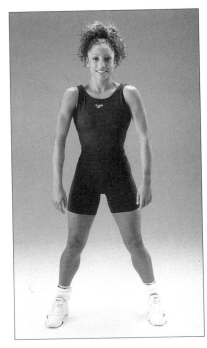

Alternate Reach Up ▼

Reach up with alternate arms (4 counts each arm). Take care not to arch the spine.

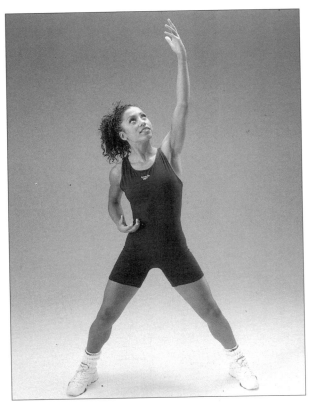
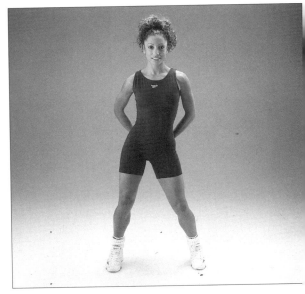

Hip Circles ▲

Circle the hips in one direction (4 counts), then repeat in the opposite direction. Keep the knees bent and don't sink into the hips.

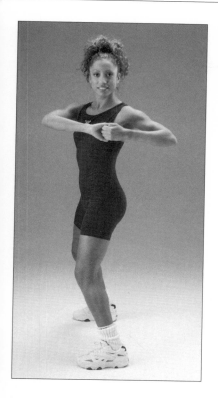

Waist Turns ◄

Keep the hips square and gently turn the shoulders but don't go beyond the full range of movement (2 counts). Keep the knees bent but don't let them roll in. Repeat to alternate sides.

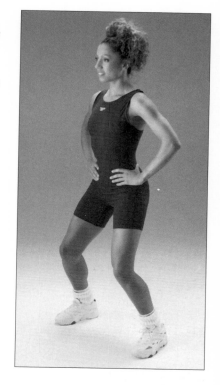

Knee Bends ►

Keep the knees over the toes throughout. Don't let them roll in towards each other. Take 2 counts down and 2 counts up.

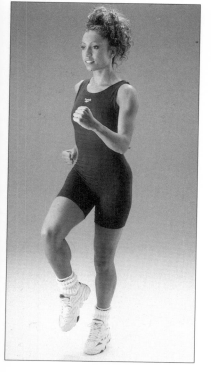

March on the spot ◄

Keep your posture upright and land through to the heels – lightly (1 count).

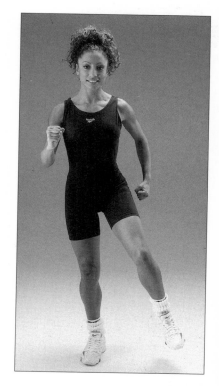

March feet apart ►

Don't stamp your feet or stick your buttocks out as you march (1 count).

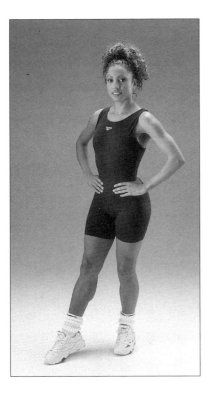

Alternate Toe Touches Front ◄

Touch alternate toes in front (2 counts each foot). Don't forget your posture.

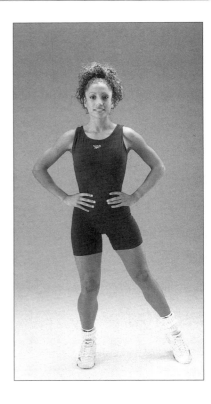

Alternate Toe Touches Side ►

Touch alternate toes to the side (2 counts each foot). Don't let the knees roll in.

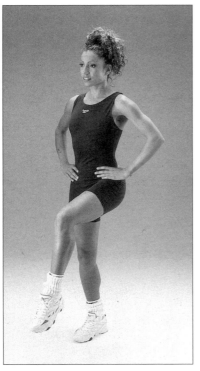

Alternate Knees Up Front ◄

Don't stick your buttocks out as you lift the knee but pull up out of the hips. Repeat with alternate knees, taking 2 counts each knee.

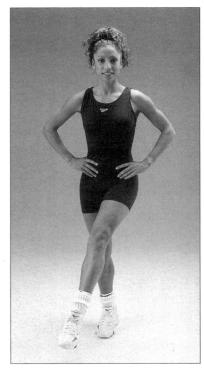

Alternate Cross Kicks Front ►

Keep these low but strong and don't lean back. Repeat with alternate legs, taking 2 counts each leg.

Alternate Side Kicks ▶

Don't throw the posture out or lift the leg too high. Repeat to alternate sides, taking 2 counts each leg.

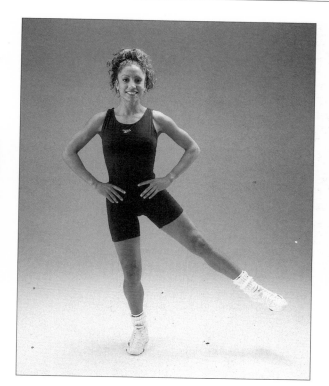

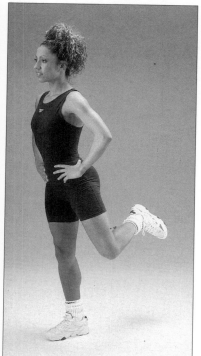

Alternate Heel Kicks to Buttocks ▲

Kick alternate heels towards your buttocks (2 counts each leg). Remember your posture.

Hopscotch Low ▶

Proceed as for Heel Kicks to Buttocks (2 counts each leg) but add a knee bend in between each kick.

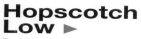

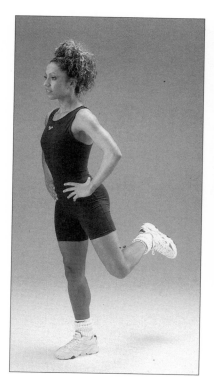

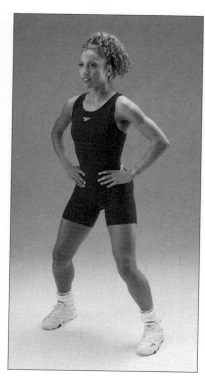

Low Jacks ▼

Stand feet together. Step to one side straight into a knee bend. Step feet together again (4 counts in all) and repeat to the other side. Check knee alignment, and don't arch the spine.

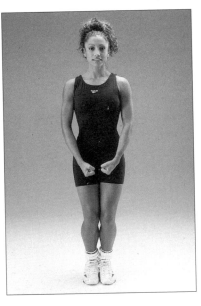 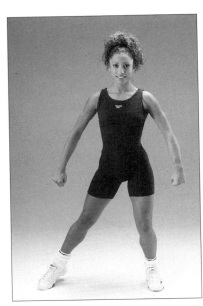 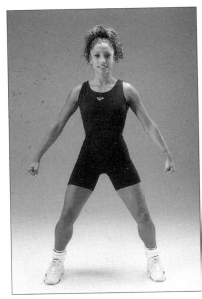

Alternate Turning Lunges ▼

Check your knees are in line with your toes and take your hips all the way round. Don't twist the knees. Repeat to alternate sides (2 counts each), bringing the feet together between each lunge.

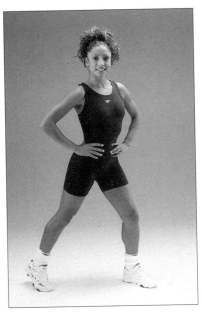 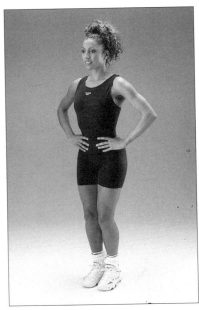 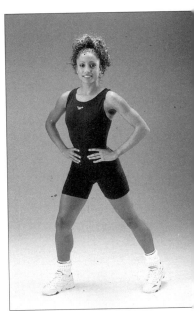

Narrow Squats ▶

Push back with your buttocks as if trying to sit on a chair. Go as low as you can, but keep the hips above the knees. Take 2 counts down, 2 counts up. Keep your stomach pulled in and don't arch the spine or hunch the shoulders.

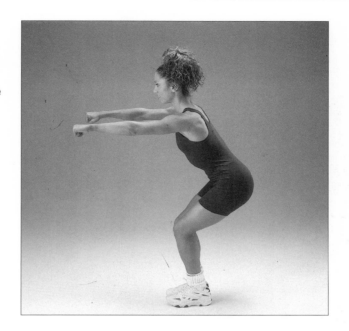

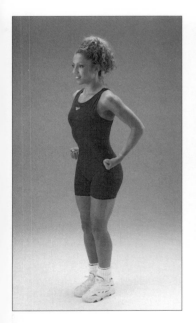
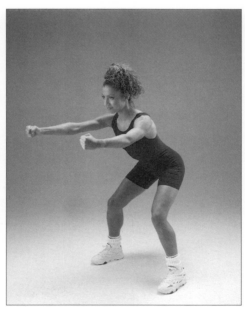
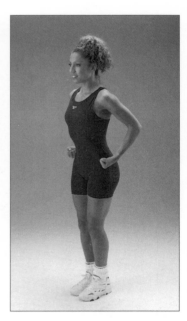

Wide Squats ▲

Step to the side with knees over toes and push back with the buttocks as with the Narrow Squat, keeping the spine straight. Bring the feet back together before stepping out to the other side. Take 2 counts down and 2 counts up.

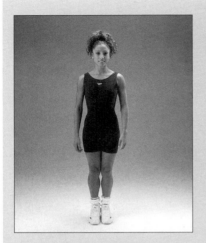 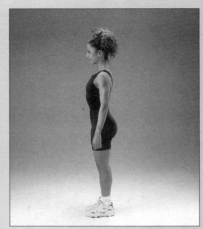 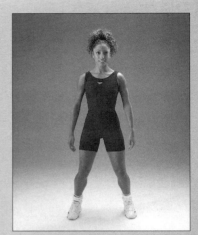

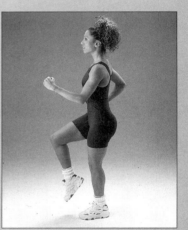

Technique Tips

✦ Check your posture (see above left and centre).

✦ Make sure your knees are in line with your toes at all times and keep the knees slightly bent to relieve pressure on the lower back.

✦ Don't let the knees roll in towards each other on the knee bends – keep them over the toes (see above right).

✦ Don't stamp when you march. Land lightly – you should not be able to hear your feet touch the floor.

✦ Don't stick your buttocks out when marching or performing the knee lifts. Instead, pull up out of the hips and, if necessary, don't lift the knees so high (see right).

The Basic Workout

Format	Approximate time
Warm-up and stretch	5 minutes
Aerobics routines	15 minutes
Cool-down and stretch	2–3 minutes
Strengthening	4 minutes
Final stretch	4 minutes
Relaxation	optional

Warm-up and Stretch

Music speed: 125–135 bpm

Warm-up I: Pulse Raiser

Approximate time: 1 minute

Exercise		Counts each	Total counts
	March on the spot × 16	1	16
	Alternate Toe Touches Front × 8	2	16
	March feet apart × 8	1	8
	March feet together × 8	1	8

Exercise		Counts each	Total counts
	Alternate Knees Up Front × 8	2	16
	March on the spot × 8	1	8
	Alternate Knees Up Front × 8	2	16
	March feet apart × 8	1	8

Warm up I continued

Exercise		Counts each	Total counts
	Alternate Heel Kicks to Buttocks x 8	2	16
	March on the spot x 8	1	8
	March feet apart x 8	1	8

Repeat Warm-up I once more (2 minutes).

Warm-up II: Limber Up

Approximate time: 1 minute
Start by standing with feet apart, knees slightly bent and in line with the toes.

Exercise	Counts each	Total counts
Shoulder Rolls Backward x 4	4	16
Shoulder Rolls Forward x 4	4	16
Alternate Reach Up x 4	4	16
Hip Circles x4	4	16

Exercise	Counts each	Total counts
Waist Turns x 8 (4 each side)	2	16
Knee Bends x 4	4	16
March on the spot x 16	1	16
Alternate Toe Touches Front x 8	2	16

Repeat Warm-up II once more (2 minutes). You should now be feeling warm and slightly out of breath. If not, repeat Warm-up I and/or II.

Warm-up III: Stretch It Out

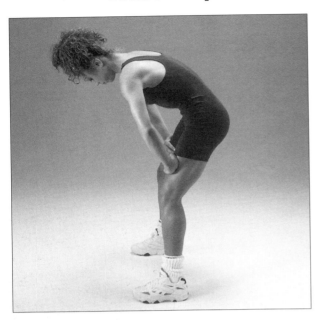
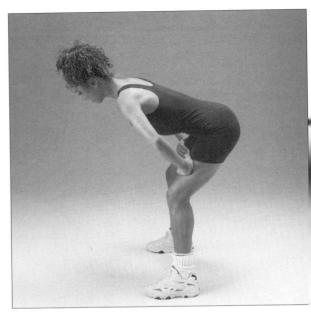

1. Lower Back Stretch ▲

Slide your hands down until they rest on your thighs. Keep the knees bent, pull your stomach in, and round your back, hunching your shoulders. Hold for 8 counts. Now, flatten out your back so that the spine and neck are in a straight line, horizontal to the floor and hold for 8 counts. Repeat each stretch once more.

2. Hamstring Stretch ▶

Slide one foot out in front of you and rest the heel on the floor. Keep your hands on your thighs for balance, but don't press down. Keep the supporting knee bent and lean forward, keeping the spine straight, until you feel a stretch up the back of the thigh of the extended leg. Don't lock out the knee. Hold for 16 counts, then change legs and repeat. Repeat once more on each side, then slowly roll up.

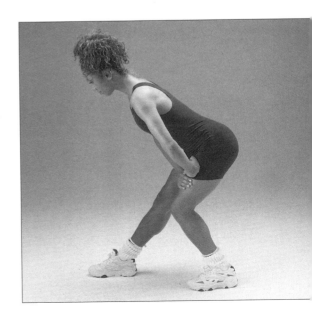

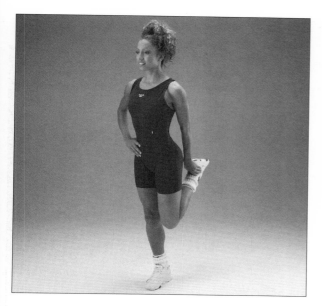

3. Quadricep Stretch ◄

Use a chair or wall for support if necessary. Lift one heel to your buttocks, keeping your knees together and slightly bending the supporting knee. Hold the ankle (not the toe) and gently pull your heel towards your buttocks and, at the same time, tilt your pelvis backward (your pubic bone forward). You should feel a stretch down the front of the thigh and across the front of the hip. Hold for 16 counts, then change legs and repeat. Make sure your posture stays upright throughout.

4. Shin Stretch ▼

Rest the front of your left foot on the floor behind you and bend both knees, gently pushing the back foot into the floor. Keep the upper body upright. Hold for 16 counts, then change feet and repeat.

For an advanced version of this stretch, rest the front of one foot on the floor in front. Bending the knees, gently push the foot into the floor (you may find this easier without shoes).

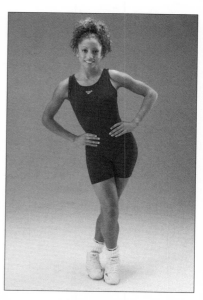

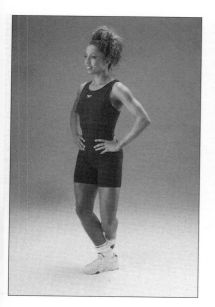

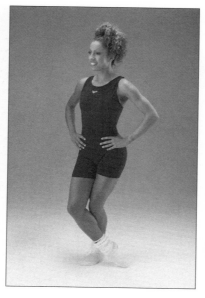

5. Outer Thigh Stretch ▲

Cross the left leg in front of the right, keeping both feet flat on the floor and knees very slightly bent. Then lean the upper body to the left, pushing your weight into the right hip. Hold for 16 counts, then change legs and repeat.

Don't hold your breath when performing the stretches. Breathe normally throughout.

6. Inner Thigh Stretch ▶

Stand with the feet apart, toes facing front and knees slightly bent. Take the weight over to the left leg, extending the right leg. Bend a little deeper or until you feel a stretch along the inside of the right leg. Hold for 16 counts, then change legs and repeat.

7. Calf Stretch ▼

Keep the feet apart and turn to face the side. Bend the front knee and extend the back leg until you feel a slight stretch in the calf. Keep both feet flat on the floor and knees in line with the toes. Hold for 16 counts. Then bend the back knee, still keeping the heel on the floor. You should feel the stretch move further down the calf. Hold for 16 counts. Change legs and stretch out the other calf.

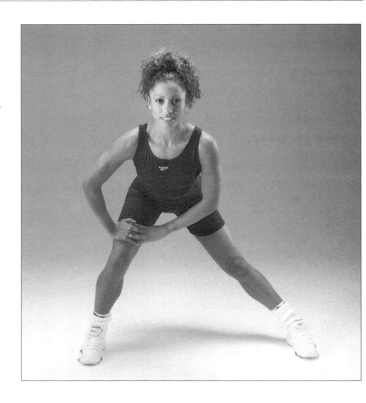

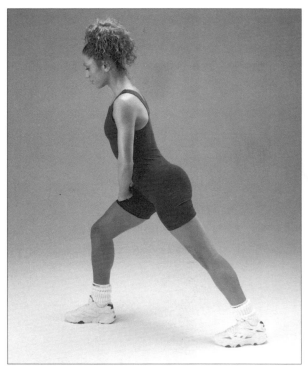

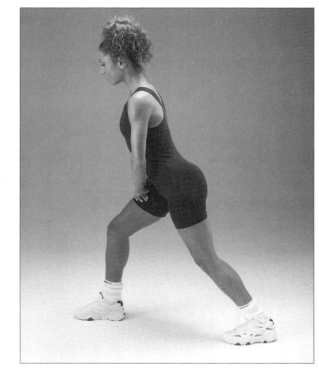

Aerobics Routines

Music speed: 128—140 bpm
Each routine lasts one minute, but repeat as indicated for optimum effect.

Aerobics Routine 1

Approximate time: 1 minute

Exercise	Counts each	Total counts
March on the spot x 16	1	16
March feet apart x 16	1	16
March feet together x 16	1	16
March feet apart x 8	1	8
March feet together x 8	1	8
March feet apart x 4	1	4
March feet together x 4	1	4
March feet apart x 4	1	4
March feet together x 4	1	4
March feet apart x 2	1	2
March feet together x 2	1	2
March feet apart x 4	1	4
March feet together x 8	1	8
Alternate Knees Up Front x 8	2	16
Alternate Toe Touches Front x 8	2	16

Repeat Routine 1 once more for all levels (2 minutes).

Aerobics Routine 2

Approximate time: 1 minute

Exercise	Counts each	Total counts
***Alternate Toe Touches Side** x 8	2	16
***Alternate Turning Lunges** x 8	2	16
***March on the spot** x 8	1	8
***Low Jacks** x 8	4	32
***March on the spot** x 8	1	8
Narrow Squats x 8	4	32
***March on the spot** x 16	1	16

Repeat Routine 2 once more for all levels (2 minutes).

Aerobics Routine 3

Approximate time: 1 minute

Exercise	Counts each	Total counts
*Alternate Knees Up Front x 8	2	16
*Alternate Heel Kicks to Buttocks x 8	2	16
*Hopscotch Low x 8	2	16
*Alternate Cross Kicks Front x 8	2	16
*Alternate Side Kicks x 8	2	16
*March feet apart x 8	1	8
Wide Squats x 8	4	32
*March on the spot x 8	1	8

For 15 minutes of aerobic work, repeat Routine 3 twice more (2 minutes), then continue as follows:

Repeat Routine 1 once

Repeat Routine 2 three times

Repeat Routine 3 three times

Repeat Routine 1 once

> Always start and finish with Routine 1 to give yourself a gentle start and wind-down to the aerobics section.

Increasing the Challenge

For a more challenging workout for those who can cope with it, add jump, skips and hops to any of the moves you feel comfortable with. The moves in Aerobics Routines 2 and 3 marked with an asterisk (*) adapt well to high-impact versions. Don't add impact to all three routines but keep Routine 1 as a respite!

Safety

Adding Impact

Marching: Marching becomes a run on the spot.

Knees Up: Add a hop.

Side and Cross Kicks: Add a hop (hop, kick).

Hopscotch Low: Add a hop and a two-footed jump (hop feet together, jump feet apart).

Heel Kicks to Buttocks: Add a two-footed jump in between kicks.

Turning Lunges: Add a jump.

Low Jacks: Add a jump.

Here are some basic rules to follow when adding high-impact moves.

✦ Do remember to wear proper shoes with plenty of cushioning.

✦ Don't work on rugs or slippery floors.

✦ Build up slowly – alternate low-impact moves with high-impact ones

✦ Limit the number of turning jumps to eight.

✦ Make sure you do the same number of jumps on each leg.

✦ Bend the knees deeper to prepare for the jumps.

✦ Land lightly with knees bent over the toes.

✦ If you find yourself landing so heavily that you can hear the noise go back to the low-impact moves until you build up more strength.

✦ Land toe, ball, heel – in that order. Always put your heels down when you land.

Cool-down and Stretch

1. Repeat Warm-up II once

2. Repeat all the stretches from the Warm-up, but hold each for six to ten counts.

Strengthening

The following upper body and trunk exercises have been chosen to complement the aerobics routines in the Basic Workout and other programmes which focus largely on the lower body.

These are best performed without music so that you can work at a pace that is comfortable for you. Otherwise, select music with approximately 120–125 beats per minute (or slower if you prefer).

Select the level of exercise appropriate to your ability. Whichever level you choose, always finish with the appropriate stretches.

If you experience any joint pain at any point during these exercises, stop immediately and consult your GP.

Abdominal Strengtheners
Preparation

Lie on your back with your knees bent and feet flat on the floor about hip-distance apart. Your pelvis should be in a neutral position. To find neutral use the 'rock and roll' test: rock the hips forward to get an exaggerated arch in the spine, then roll the hips down to push the lower back into the floor. Now let the pelvis rest between these two positions. Pull your stomach in to stabilize the spine and pelvis.

In the following abdominal exercises, exhale as you lift up, and inhale as you lower down to the floor.

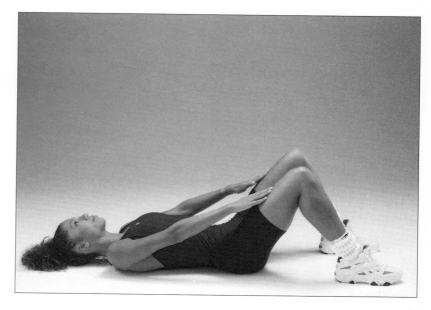

Level 1: Absolute Beginners

Abdomen ►

Slide your hands up your thighs so that your shoulders lift off the floor. Lift up on 4 counts, and lower on 4 counts. Control the lowering so that your shoulders don't touch the floor until count four. If necessary, gently hold on to your thighs as you lower until you have built up sufficient strength. Repeat 4 times. Then repeat an additional 8 times lifting on 2 counts, and lowering on 2 counts.

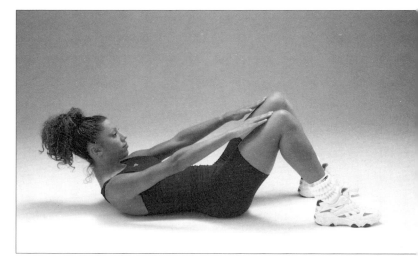

Waist ►

Slide both hands up one knee, lifting on 4 counts, and lowering on 4 counts. Repeat on the other side, then repeat once more on each side. Control the lowering, and don't arch the spine. Keep the neck long and don't scrunch the chin into the chest.

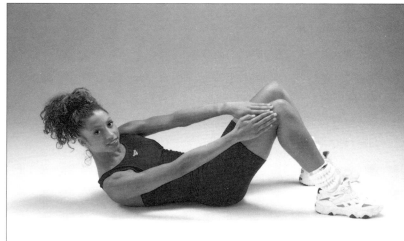

Level 2: Beginners

Do the Level 1 exercises plus the following:

Abdomen ◄

Place your hands across your chest and lift the shoulders off the floor on 2 counts, then lower on 2 counts. Repeat 8 times, rest, then repeat a further 8 times.

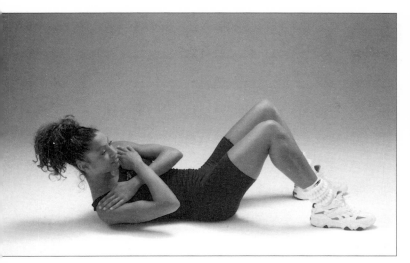

Waist ◄

Keeping your hands on your chest, lift the shoulders diagonally towards one knee on 2 counts, and lower on 2 counts. Repeat, lifting towards the other knee. Repeat 8 times, rest, then repeat a further 8 times.

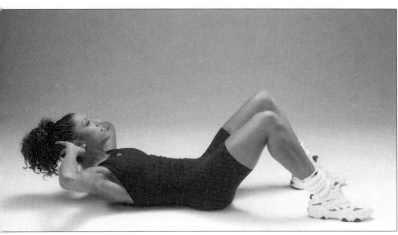

Level 3: Intermediate

Do the Level 2 exercises plus the following:

Abdomen ◄

Place your fingertips on your earlobes. Keeping your elbows pushed back in line with the shoulders, lift up on 2 counts, and lower on 2 counts. Look up at the ceiling and don't pull on your head or neck. Repeat 8 times, rest, then repeat a further 8 times.

Waist ►

Lift your legs and cross them at the ankles. Make sure your pelvis remains in a neutral position. With your fingertips on your earlobes, lift the shoulders as before, then take one shoulder towards the opposite knee. Lift up on 2 counts, and lower on 2 counts. Repeat, taking the other shoulder towards the opposite knee. Repeat 8 times, then rest and repeat a further 8 times.

Level 4: Intermediate Plus and above

Proceed as for Level 3 but repeat each exercise in sets of 8 repetitions.

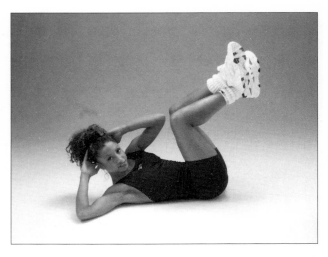

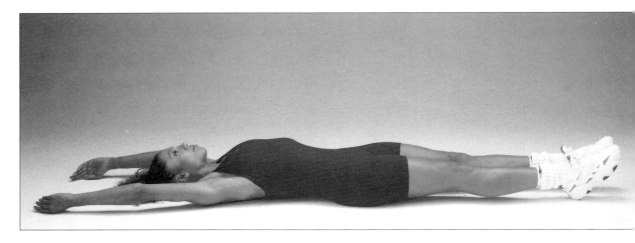

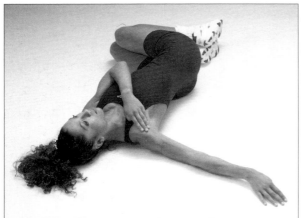

Abdominal Stretch

(All levels) ▲
Stretch your legs out and stretch your arms above your head. Hold until you feel the tension in your abdomen release.

◄ Now, bend the knees up and let them fall to one side of your body while stretching your arms to the opposite side. Hold until the tension releases, then change sides and repeat.

Chest and Arm Strengtheners
Preparation ►

Place a cushion or rolled towel under your knees, and position yourself on all fours, with hands shoulder-width apart and knees hip-distance apart.

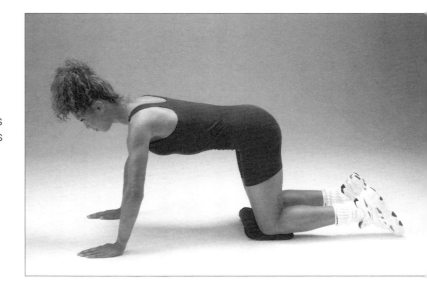

Level 1: Absolute Beginners ▶

Keeping your back straight, lower your upper body to the floor but keep your buttocks in the air (make sure the curtains are drawn!). Your nose should touch the floor, but don't arch your spine or hunch your shoulders. Take 4 counts to go down and 4 to come up. Repeat 8 times, rest then repeat a further 8 times.

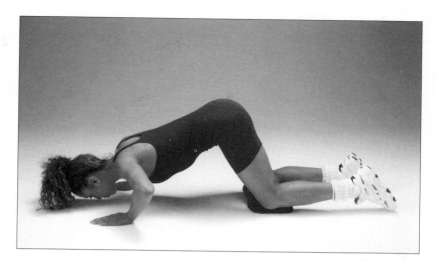

Level 2: Beginners

Proceed as for Level 1, but faster. Take 2 counts to go down and 2 to come up. Repeat 16 times, rest, then repeat a further 16 times.

Level 3: Intermediate ▶

Move your hands further forward but keep them shoulder-width apart. Keep your back straight but lengthening away from your legs. Now, aim to get your chest on the floor by moving the body in one unit – don't leave your buttocks in the air or arch your spine. Neither your nose nor your tummy should touch the floor. Take 2 counts to go down and 2 to come up. Repeat 16 times, rest, then repeat a further 16 times.

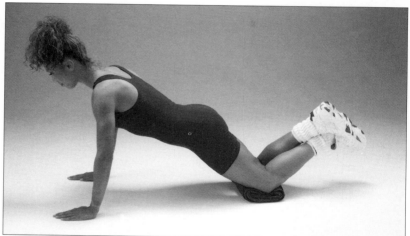

Level 4: Intermediate Plus and above

Proceed as for Level 3, and repeat until you fatigue.

Note: **The full press-up from the toes should only be attempted by very strong individuals.**

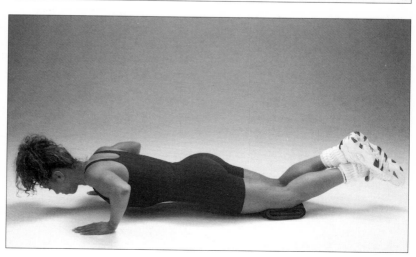

Chest Stretch

(All levels) ▼

Kneel back on your haunches and stretch your arms out along the floor. Hold until the tension releases.

► Move to a sitting position and clasp both hands behind your back. Pull your hands away from you to stretch out the chest. Hold until the tension releases.

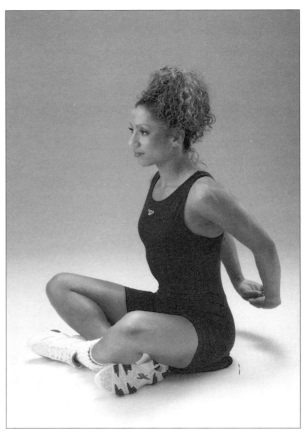

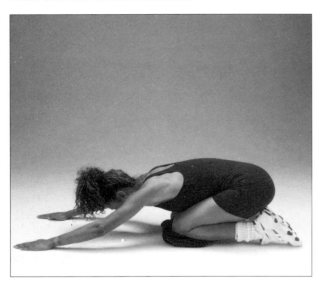

Final Stretch

Music speed: 90–100 bpm
The first three stretches can also be performed standing, or sitting on a chair. For the remaining (lying) stretches use cushions or towels where needed.

Back Stretch ►

Clasp your hands in front of you, with palms facing away. Push away with your hands and lean backward slightly to stretch out the neck and shoulders. Hold until the tension releases.

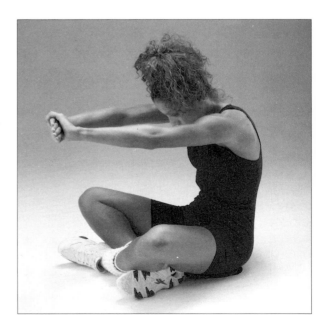

Side Stretch ▶

Place one hand on the floor for support. Keeping your back straight, stretch up to the ceiling and over your head with the other arm. Feel the stretch down the side of your body. Hold until the tension releases, then repeat to the other side.

Spine Stretch ▼

Sitting cross-legged, place your hands gently on the back of your head and let your head drop forward. Lean backward until you feel a stretch up the spine. Hold until the tightness lessens, then sit up straight.

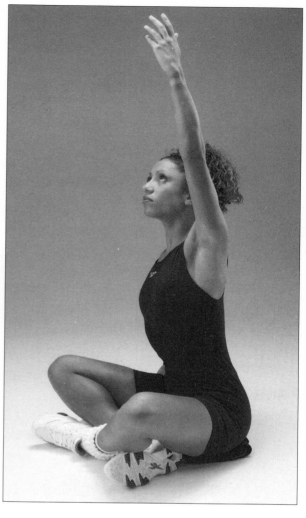

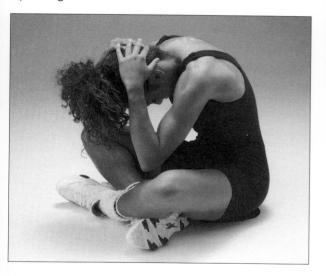

Hip Stretch ◀

Lie on your back, bend your knees up and cross one foot over the other knee. Pull the underneath leg towards the body until you feel a tightness in the hip and buttock area. Hold until the tightness lessens, then change legs and repeat.

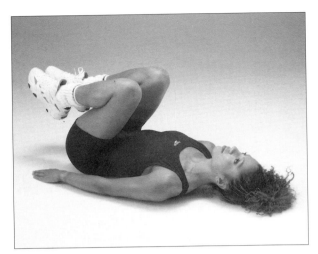

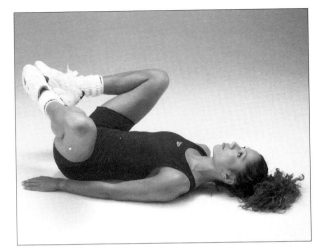

Inner Thigh Stretch ▲

Bend both knees in towards your chest and let them fall apart until you feel tension in the inner thigh and groin area. Hold until the tension releases.

► For an advanced version of this stretch, repeat as above but with legs extended.

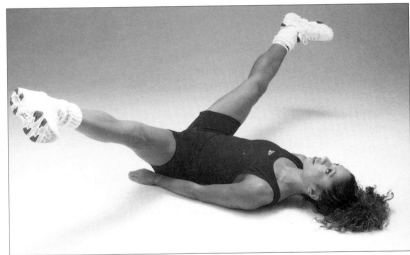

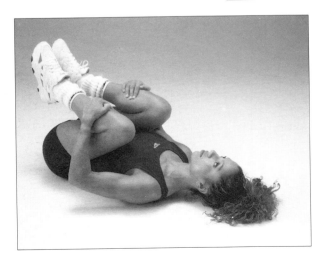

◄ Lower Back Stretch

Hug both knees to your chest until you feel tension in the lower spine. Hold until the tension releases.

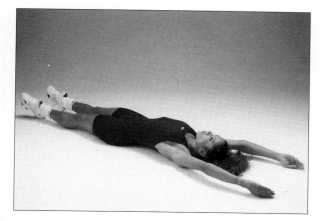

Relaxation

Turn off the music or put on one of your favourite soothing romantic tracks, and turn the lights down low.

Lie on the floor on your back and stretch out from top to toe, as if trying to push your hands into an imaginary wall beyond your head and your toes into the 'wall' beyond your feet.

Stretch as hard as you can for a few seconds, then release completely and flop 'into' the floor and enjoy the contrasting sensation of relaxation. Repeat twice more.

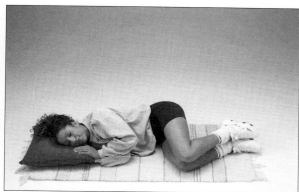

Put on a sweatshirt and snuggle down on a rug or blanket, resting your head on a pillow or cushion. Make sure you are comfortable and close your eyes for five minutes or until the end of the music track. Use this time to focus on pleasant images – or on absolutely nothing if you are able to do that. Don't worry if you drift off into a snooze – this is what it's about. When your time is up (it's useful to have an alarm clock for this, but not an 'angry' bell – use one of the more gentle electronic ones), move very slowly – don't jump up suddenly.

Getting Up Technique

Use the following technique to get up off the floor from a lying or sitting position without straining your back.

Roll onto your side (as above). Move on to all fours, then come up on to one knee, using your hands for support. Place your hands on your knee and push yourself up to a standing position, then slowly uncurl the spine.

Well done! You have just completed your first workout.

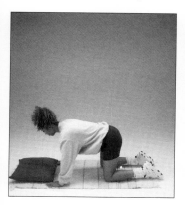
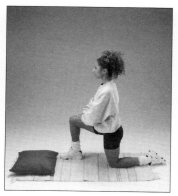
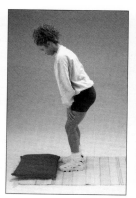
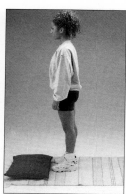

Walk Reebok

The Walk Reebok training programme is perhaps the simplest of all the programmes in that it needs the minimum of equipment and can be carried out almost anywhere and at any time, providing certain provisos for safety are followed.

But don't make the mistake of thinking walking is an easy option. It is now recognized as a bona fide exercise programme with important health and fitness benefits and can be a useful aid to weight loss. It is also used by many top athletes and sports people to complement their regular training.

Simplicity is the secret of its success. Because walking is a relatively simple activity, people tend to do it more often and for far longer than they would any other form of exercise. The end result is that they accumulate a greater number of exercise sessions per week and, consequently, achieve far better results.

What is Walk Reebok?

The principle behind the Walk Reebok training programme is that it takes a form of physical activity that most people already do and hones your posture and walking technique in such a way that you can comfortably walk for greater distances or at greater speeds. It's not a question of teaching you how to walk, but how to walk better and for greater fitness benefits.

What Does It Involve?

Like all the other Reebok training programmes, Walk Reebok is a complete exercise format, with warm-up and cool-down guidelines and a customized aerobics section that can be tailored to your individual fitness level and exercise needs. It can also be performed indoors on a treadmill.

Walk Reebok is based on three techniques. The first is the basic, introductory technique that focuses on improving posture and walking style. The second technique aims to refine the moves slightly and allows for an increase in intensity. The third concentrates on a very distinctive development of the technique which allows the participant to substantially increase the intensity of their workout.

The three techniques can be intermingled to form a challenging, but achievable, interval workout that is fun to do. You'll enjoy this new efficient way of walking so much that you'll be using it as you rush around the supermarket trying to get to the checkout before the crowds.

What Will It Do For Me?

Walking has both health and fitness benefits. Simply to get out in the fresh air and take part in some regular activity is particularly good for the overstressed, overweight, inactive or the reluctant exerciser. 'Time out' on your own, away from the office or demands of family life is an excellent anti-stress measure and a natural by-product of a quick stroll around the park. On the other hand, if you build up the pace a little and gradually start walking specific distances or for specific lengths of time on a regular basis, you will soon develop a very effective, easy-to-maintain fitness programme.

Walk Reebok: The Benefits

✦ Carries the same cardiovascular benefits as other aerobic activities.
✦ A low-impact activity with a low injury potential.
✦ A good calorie-burner.
✦ Can be a useful aid to weight loss.
✦ Tones the thighs and buttocks.
✦ Improves balance, coordination and agility.
✦ Improves posture.
✦ Helps lower the risk of heart disease.
✦ Can contribute to an increase in bone density.
✦ Easy to do and easy to maintain.
✦ Suits all ages and abilities.

Factfile

Just five 30-minute walking sessions of approximately two miles each per week can reduce the risk of heart attack by more than 25 per cent.

A ten-and-a-half-stone person walking at three and a half miles an hour will burn approximately 300 calories per hour.

Where to Start

One of the advantages of walking is that the intensity level is self-dictated. In other words, there is no set speed or distance to begin with. You start off at your own natural pace and as your fitness level and ability increases, you 'up' the pace accordingly.

However, most people have developed poor posture habits over the years, and poor posture and technique can lead to injuries. So whether you intend to follow this programme alone or join a walking group, it's always a good idea to get these checked out first. As with all Reebok® programmes there is a hotline number that you can call to find a Walk Reebok instructor or walking group near you (see back of book for details). You don't have to attend all the sessions if you are a convicted lone exerciser, but do use the instructor's expert eye to give your walking style and habits the once over to ensure you are walking as efficiently and safely as possible.

How to Start

Aim to start out with just short walks to begin with. Consider how you might incorporate these into your everyday life. If you live fairly near your place of work, perhaps you could plan to walk part of the way and then gradually build up over the weeks so that you can walk the full distance there and back.

Alternatively, select times of the day when you could spend 15 to 20 minutes walking. Start out at a comfortable pace, using Walk Reebok Technique 1, and build up to three times a week. When you feel comfortable with this, increase the pace and alter the technique so that you gradually start walking a greater part of the distance, using Walk Reebok Technique 2. Once this becomes comfortable, try adding another day's walking, ideally targeting five to six days a week. But don't alter the speed or the distance. Remember, change only one element at a time.

So, for a complete beginner the start-up programme could look like this:

Beginner's Start-up Plan

	Frequency	Intensity	Duration
Week 1	twice	Technique 1	10–15 minutes
Week 2	two to three times	Technique	10–15 minutes
Week 3	three times	Technique 1	15–20 minutes
Week 4	three times	Technique 1/2	20 minutes
Week 5	three times	Technique 1/2	20–25 minutes
Week 6	three times	Technique 1/2	25 minutes

Note how Technique 2 is not brought in until week 4. Some people may find they can move up sooner, while others will need a slower introduction to activity of any nature. Equally, Technique 2 may only take up a few minutes of each session, so you can alternate between Techniques 1 and 2 as you feel able. The overall aim is to build up the intensity, frequency and duration to a level where training benefits are achieved. Once this becomes comfortable, you may continue as follows for the next six weeks.

	Frequency	Intensity	Duration
Week 7	four times	Technique 1/2	25 minutes
Week 8	four times	Technique 1/2	25–30 minutes
Week 9	four times	Technique 1/2/3*	25–30 minutes
Week 10	five times	Technique 1/2/3*	30–35 minutes
Week 11	five times	Technique 1/2/3*	30–35 minutes
Week 12	five times	Technique 1/2/3*	35+ minutes

*Introducing Technique 3 at this stage is optional and should be built in gradually. To begin with, walk at this pace for one minute only, alternating with Techniques 1 and 2.

If you chose to build up speed and frequency as above in the first twelve weeks, the next phase could be to go out for longer walks. At first you might need to decrease the speed a little on longer walks in order to maintain the endurance, but once your body becomes acclimatized to the change you can soon build up the speed again. Remember, Technique 3 can be interspersed with Techniques 1 and 2. You don't have to walk the whole session at high speeds, but the aim is to develop a brisk speed over most of the walk.

Speed Versus Distance

Increasing either the speed or distance is a good way of making your 'walkout' more effective. Select according to your personal timetable and fitness level. You can intermingle the two, but don't try to increase both at the same time. For example, you may choose to do frequent but short, fast walks during the week and go for a longer, less hasty walk on the weekend when you perhaps have more time.

How Fast or Slow?

It is also important to note that what may be a fast speed for one person may not feel so arduous for another. So be sure to walk at the correct pace for you. However, in order for your walk to be effective, you need to do more than just 'window shop'. While the occasional stroll is very relaxing, it will not offer fitness training benefits unless it keeps you at a slightly breathy pitch for at least 15 consecutive minutes.

Technique 1 could be discribed as a continuous (15–20 minutes) comfortable strolling pace. Technique 2 is a more brisk pace, and Technique 3 is a fast walk – imagine you are rushing for a bus or late for an appointment. As you learn the techniques you'll be surprised how soon you will be able to walk even faster.

Factors Affecting Intensity

✦ **Hills** You can also increase the intensity of your workout by increasing the number and steepness of the hills you include in your route. Progress gradually and plan your route carefully so that the inclines are not too steep or too many for you to comfortably climb. If possible, aim to hit a hill at least ten minutes into your walk when your body will be warm but not too fatigued. However, don't add hills to your route until you are competent at the technique you have chosen to do. Ensure you tackle big hills at a manageable speed – you are already increasing the intensity by going up the hill, and you want to reach the top and live to see another day!

Arm Movements The faster you move your arms, the faster you will walk and the more demanding the walk becomes. However, keep the arm movements restricted to the natural swing described in the technique section in order not to compromise your posture.

Weights The natural weight of your body, arms and legs will give sufficient resistance to offer some muscle toning. If you want to increase your muscular strength and endurance, use weights at a separate session or when you have finished walking but *not* while walking. Otherwise, using weights may compromise your posture and technique.

Duration and Frequency

Remember, how often, how hard, how far and how fast you walk are all important elements to consider if you want to achieve fitness benefits. But increase only one element at a time in order to prevent overuse injury or fatigue.

Planning Tips

Beginners: Plan your route along flat ground only.

Intermediate: When you become more experienced add a few undulating routes to your regular walks, but always allow sufficient level ground in order for you to 'recover'.

Advanced: Include any hills that you can cope with, but pay attention to your 'climbing' technique, and slow down to a manageable pace to tackle the big ones.

Balancing Your Programme

Remember to balance the workload on your body each week by alternating the type of workouts you do and allowing for some rest time. You may choose to use Walk Reebok as your main form of exercise, or you may use it to complement one of the other programmes. If you choose Walk Reebok as your main activity, your weekly schedule could look like the one below (this assumes you have been using Walk Reebok Technique 3 for some time).

Suggested Weekly Schedule

Monday	Walk Reebok	1 hour	Technique 1/2/3
Tuesday	Swim	1 hour	Gentle
Wednesday	Walk Reebok	1 hour	Technique 1/2/3
Thursday	Rest		
Friday	Walk Reebok	1 hour	Technique 1/2/3
Saturday	Badminton	1 hour	Fairly hard
Sunday	Walk Reebok	2 hours	Technique 1/2

Safety Tips for Walking

◆ Always try to walk with a partner.
◆ If you must walk alone, let a friend or neighbour know your route and estimated walking time. If there is no one to tell, leave a note inside your home in a visible place.
◆ Stick to familiar neighbourhoods with plenty of activity.
◆ Know your route. When travelling, ask the staff at the hotel desk for safe walking routes, and advise them of your plans.
◆ Varying your route prevents boredom and promotes safety. Never let your route become predictable to others.
◆ Try to walk in the daylight. Remember, the darkness before sunrise can harbour the same dangers as the darkness after sunset. If you must walk in the dark, choose a well-lit path and wear reflective clothing so you are visible to motorists.
◆ If you feel that you are being followed by a motor vehicle, turn around and walk the other way, remaining on the same side of the road.
◆ Walk in the middle of pavements rather than close to alleyways, buildings or parked cars.
◆ Never wear expensive jewellery or carry valuables when walking.
◆ Observe your environment without distractions. Never use a personal stereo during your walk.
◆ Trust your instinct when it tells you something feels unsafe. Turn around, cross the street, or go for help.
◆ Stay alert, aware and in control. Radiate confidence and purpose.

Record Your Progress

◆ Use the walking log on page 156 to keep a record of your route and monitor how hard you worked. As the weeks go by, check back to see how much you have progressed.

◆ Time your walk and make a note of it on the log. Use a pedometer as you walk or take the car out and measure the approximate distance you walked. Look back at your progress over the weeks and see how much quicker you now walk the same distance.

Walk Reebok Technique

Posture Check ▶

Before learning the techniques, check your posture to ensure you stand and walk correctly. Stand tall with shoulders back and down, chest open and chin in. Keep the shoulders level, the knees and hips straight and the pelvis in a neutral position.

Walk Reebok Technique 1

Approximate speed range: 16–30 minutes per mile

The aim is to maintain good posture and techniqueand a comfortable pace. Check out the following:

1. Arm Action ▼

The arms should swing from the shoulders, not the elbows, and the swing should feel natural and comfortable. The arms should swing in opposition to the legs and should not cross the centre of the body. Don't let the elbows stick out.

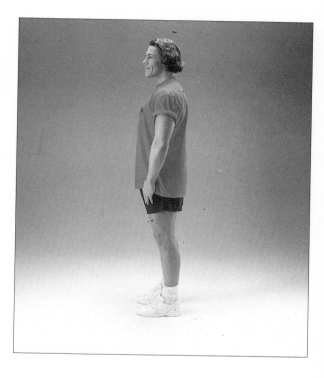

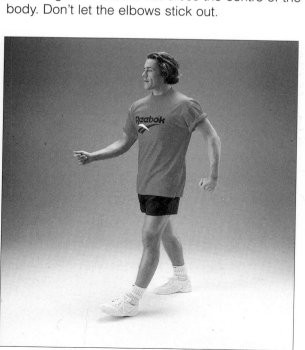

2. Leg Action ◀

The length of your stride should be comfortable, and the legs should swing from the hips not the knees. Inflexibility in the hamstrings and hips may shorten the natural stride. People with short legs will generally have a shorter stride length than those with long legs.

Arm and leg action. Arm swings from the shoulder, not the elbow, and leg swings from the hip, not the knee.

81

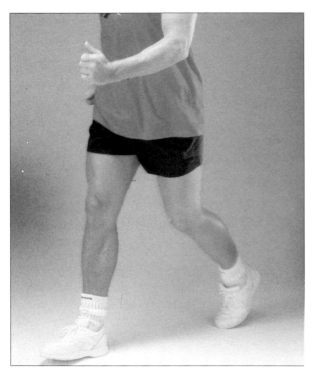

3. Foot Action ◄

The heel should strike the ground first and roll through to the ball of the foot. Both the heel strike and forefoot fall should be noiseless.

Practise Technique 1 until it feels comfortable. Although it appears simple, you'll be surprised how many bad walking habits you have picked up over the years. When you are completely comfortable with this technique and are able to maintain it for at least 20 minutes, move on to Technique 2.

Walk Reebok Technique 2

Approximate speed range: 13–15 minutes per mile

Don't forget to check your posture before you start.

1. Arm Action ◄

Speeding up the arm movement will help the legs to speed up too, so efficient arm movements are imperative. The arms will naturally bend at the elbows as you speed up, but ensure the elbows stay 'flexed' at about a 90-degree angle and that the forearms do not flop about. Make sure the arm swing still comes from the shoulders, that the arms don't swing across the body and that the elbows swing snugly past the waist. On the forward swing, the hips should not swing much higher than the chest. On the backward swing, think of pushing the elbows backward so that your fists are almost at hip level, but don't allow the hands to go behind the hips. The arms will then naturally swing forward by the right amount.

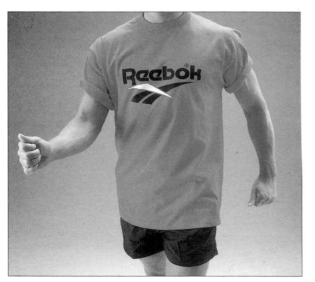

Technique tip

Make loose fists with the hands and turn the thumbs up to the ceiling – this helps to keep the arms swinging in the right direction.

2. Leg Action ▶

The back leg should be fully
extended as you walk but don't
completely lock out the knee.
Too much bend in the knee will
cause you to 'bob' up and
down, while too much 'locking'
of the knees will strain the
knees and make striding difficult. Aim for a smooth walk, and
keep your head at the same
level throughout.

**Arm and leg action. Arms are slightly
bent and tight into the waist as you
speed up. Don't lock out the back
knee.**

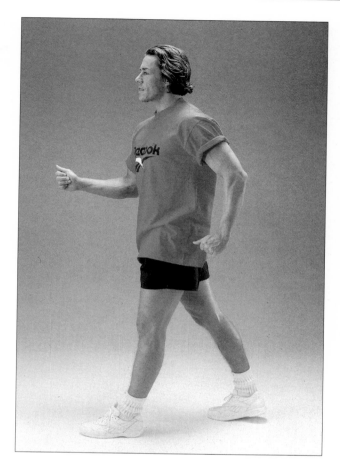

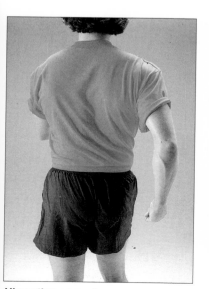

Hip action correct.

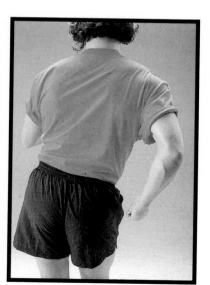

Hip action incorrect.

3. Hip Action ◀

The hips should rock forward
and back naturally. The faster
you walk, the more pronounced
this roll will become. If you
swing the legs from the hips,
this will automatically pull the
hip forward. Don't force the hip
movement but let it evolve as a
result of the walking.

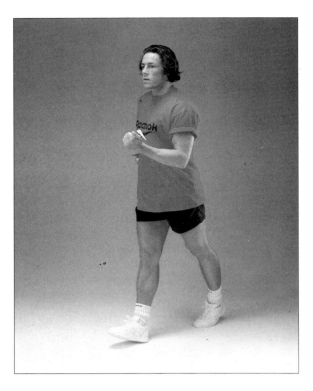

4. Foot Action ◄

Use the same foot action as Technique 1, but concentrate on pushing off the ball of the back foot and increasing the front toe raise. But don't let the toes slap down. The faster the rear leg is brought forward, the faster the rate of walking. As you speed up you will need to shorten the pace slightly.

5. Forward Lean ▶

As you speed up you will find a very slight lean starts to occur. Make sure this lean happens from the ankle not the waist.

Practise Technique 2 until you feel completely at ease and can easily speed up and slow down between Techniques 1 and 2. When you can maintain Technique 2 for at least 20 minutes, move on to Technique 3.

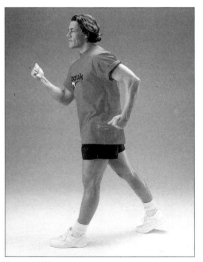

Forward lean correct.

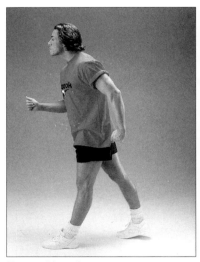

Forward lean incorrect.

Walk Reebok Technique 3

Approximate speed range: 12 minutes per mile or faster

Note: This is an advanced technique, so proceed with caution. Although you may have mastered Techniques 1 and 2, you will still find that you need a little time to acclimatize to the demands of Technique 3, so progress gradually. Remember to check your posture.

1. Arm Action ▶

Use the same arm action as Technique 2, but concentrate on a neat, tight swing and push the elbows as far back as possible, keeping the hands in line with the hips or waist. The faster the arms swing, the faster the legs will go.

2. Leg Action ▶

Now you will have to shorten your stride because you need to do more steps per minute. The leg swing should still come from the hip. Concentrate on pulling the back leg through as fast as possible.

Right: Arm and leg action. Arms are held firmly at your sides, and the stride shortens.

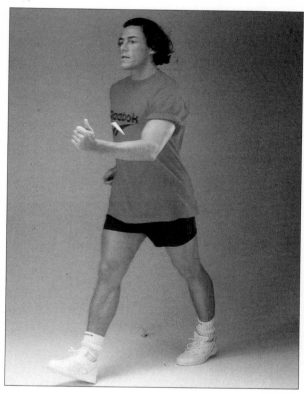

3. Hip Action

This becomes more pronounced in Technique 3. As the legs move through faster, the hips need to rotate forward and backward (not up and down). Don't wiggle the hips but let them follow the legs so that the same hip as front leg goes forward.

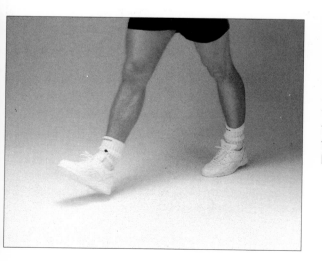

4. Foot Action ◀

The toe raise should be such that oncomers can almost see the whole of the sole of your shoe. The feet come closer together as if walking along the outside edge of a tightrope, but without crossing the feet over. This way, you can walk faster but still maintain the natural heel/toe roll of each foot.

5. Forward Lean ▶

The forward lean should still come from the ankle, not the waist, and the faster you walk the more pronounced this will be. Make sure you don't cheat by sticking out the chin. Think of leading with the chest so that if you were in a race your chest would cross the line first, but don't stick your buttocks out!

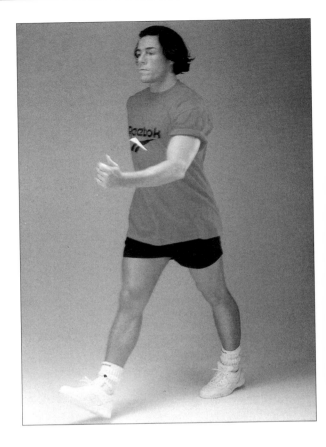

6. Hill Technique

Going up hills requires a slight alteration to the body lean. Lean into the hill, but keep upright. The steeper the incline, the more you will need to lean into the hill. You'll find that the incline of the hill will slow you down slightly, so shorten the strides even more to climb the hill without losing too much momentum. Keep your head up and look at the top of the hill.

Going down hills requires you to bend the knees more so that you can stay in control of your centre of gravity and control your speed of descent. Keep your weight over your heels and resist the temptation to lean backward. On steep hills shorten the stride again. The steeper the hill, the deeper the knee bend. Be prepared to slow down to manage the hill successfully.

Practice Makes Perfect

Practise each of the techniques until you are completely comfortable with them, and slowly build up the time spent using each one. When you feel confident, try extending the time spent walking each week. On the following pages is a simple workout format that you can follow to help build up those walking hours.

Walk Reebok: The 30-minute Walking Workout

Warm-up and Stretch

Indoors: Use the warm-up and stretch from the Basic Workout (5 minutes) plus the additional stretches below.

or

Outdoors: Use Technique 1 for 5 minutes, or until the body temperature is raised, then do the stretches from the warm-up section of the Basic Workout, plus the additional stretches below.

Upper Back Stretch ▶

Stand with feet hip-distance apart and knees slightly bent. Roll your hips back and pubic bone forward (pelvic tilt). Clasp your hands in front of your chest and push the palms away from your body. Round the shoulders and push gently until you feel the stretch across the top of your back. Hold until the tension releases, then repeat once more.

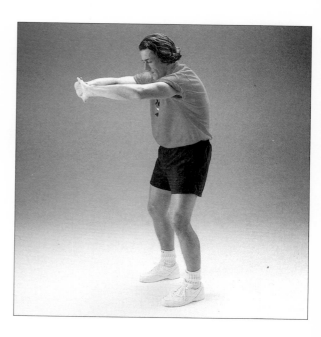

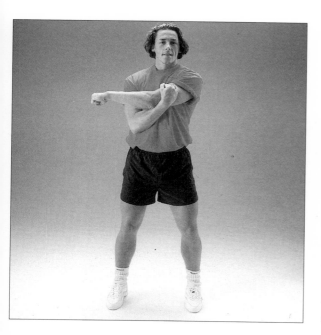

Shoulder Stretch ◀

Keep the knees slightly bent and tilt the pelvis. Cross your right arm in front of your body and wrap the left arm around it. Push away from your body with the right arm and at the same time push into your body with the left arm. The pressure of both arms pushing against each other should result in a comfortable stretch across the shoulder joint. Hold until the tension releases, then change over arms and repeat.

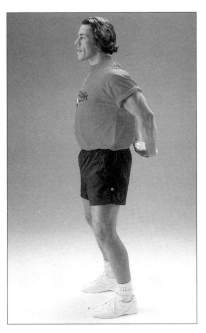

Chest Stretch ◄

Clasp your hands behind your back, with elbows slightly bent. Slowly raise the arms away from the body, and hold. You should feel the stretch across your chest. Hold until the tension releases, then release and repeat.

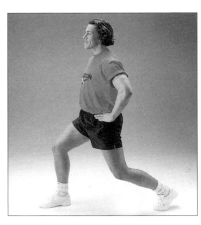

Hip Flexor Stretch ◄

Place one foot in front of the other, with knees bent and the back heel raised. Tuck the buttocks tightly under your hips while contracting the abdominals. You should feel the stretch in the front of the hip and upper thigh region of the back leg. Hold until the tension releases, then repeat on the other leg.

Aerobics Section

For 20 minutes of aerobic work proceed as follows.

	Action	Approximate time
1.	Gradually build up from Technique 1 to Technique 2	3 minutes
2.	Alternate Technique 1 with Technique 3	2 minutes
3.	Alternate Technique 1 with Technique 2	2 minutes
4.	Repeat step 3 four times	8 minutes
5.	Move back to Technique 1	5 minutes

Cool-down and Stretch

Use Technique 1 for a further 3 minutes then repeat the Upper Back, Shoulder, Chest and Hip Flexor stretches above. For the 30-minute workout, turn to page 72 for the final stretch. If you wish to add a strengthening session, turn to page 66 and follow the cool-down instructions before doing any strengthening work. Always finish with the final stretch.

The Advanced Challenge

For those who want a greater challenge, repeat the aerobics section to extend the walk, or plan a route to take in some hills, but remember your hill technique.

Step Reebok

Step Reebok® is one of the world's most popular exercise programmes, with classes taking place in over 40 countries around the globe. Based on scientific research, the Step Reebok training programme introduced one of the first types of standardized exercise with identifiable moves and a piece of equipment with measurable increments This meant that classes across the world could be standardized and similar guidelines on entry levels, safety and effectiveness set. The adjustability of the platform and the uniformity of the moves also offered the opportunity for mixed ability classes so that both men and women of all ages and abilities could enjoy a Step Reebok class.

What Is Step Reebok?

The Step Reebok® programme primarily works the major muscle groups in the legs and buttocks and is an excellent form of aerobic fitness training. The introductory programme is largely low impact and carried out relatively slowly compared to most aerobics classes. Consequently, beginners can quickly feel comfortable with the programme and are more likely to 'stick with it'.

What Does It Involve?

Essentially, it involves stepping up and down off a platform to music and incorporates a variety of leg and arm movements. The step patterns are easy to learn and do not involve any complicated 'dance-type' moves.

What Will It Do For Me?

Step Reebok can be as intense as running at 7 mph (very fast!), yet with impact forces on the body similar to walking. It is therefore a very effective form of cardiovascular training. In addition, it strengthens and tones the lower body, improves coordination skills, balance and agility and can be a useful aid to weight loss. Calories burned are subject to your own body weight (see page 157).

Step Reebok: The Benefits

✦ Forms a great aerobic workout.

✦ A low-impact but high-intensity activity.

✦ A good calorie burner.

✦ A useful aid to weight loss.

✦ Tones the thighs and buttocks.

✦ Improves balance, coordination and agility.

✦ Contains simple, uniform moves.

✦ Suits many abilities.

✦ Popular with both men and women.

Where to Start

Always start at a level appropriate to your fitness and skill ability. Newcomers to Step Reebok should aim to step on a platform height of four to six inches to begin with. Even if you are 'aerobically' fit or have strong or long legs, you should still follow these guidelines to start with, since your muscles will need time to acclimatize to this new activity. Only increase the height of the platform when you feel *completely* comfortable with all of the moves at that level. (Increasing the platform height by two inches can increase the intensity of the workload by 12 per cent – that's quite a lot over a 20-minute session.)

Platform Height Guidelines

The following are general guidelines. The length of your legs will to some extent dictate the platform height you choose. Long legs feel more comfortable on a higher platform and short legs on a lower platform. If in doubt it is always wise to start with a low platform height. Even advanced steppers with short legs may need to use a low platform height:
Beginners: 4 to 6 inches
Intermediate: 6 to 8 inches
Advanced: 8 to 10 inches

How to Start

As with all new activities, progress gradually. If you are not performing any other form of exercise, you should start with at least two sessions per week and aim to build up gradually, adding only *one* new element at a time. This way, you will increase the training benefits while keeping the injury risk to a minimum. So, if you are increasing the length of your workout or the difficulty of the moves, don't add arm movements or increase the platform height as well.

You can combine Step Reebok with complementary activities that use different body parts or offer different training benefits. Give yourself time (a couple of weeks) to acclimatize to each new change. Once you have built up to three Step Reebok sessions a week, your schedule could look something like this.

Suggested Weekly Schedule

Monday	Step Reebok	30 minutes
Tuesday	Swim or aqua aerobics	60 minutes
Wednesday	Step Reebok	30 minutes
Thursday	Rest	
Friday	Yoga or stretch class	60 minutes
Saturday	Step Reebok	30 minutes
Sunday	Rest	

Plan your weekly schedule around your own personal fitness objectives. Use the exercise schedule on page 154 to help you plan your week and chart your progress.

Factors Affecting Intensity

Step Reebok is a relatively intensive workout even on a low platform, so be sure you are comfortable with the most basic moves before progressing. It is also important to be aware of the factors that can easily affect the intensity.

Arm Movements

When arm movements are included in an activity, particularly large arm movements above shoulder level, the heart rate will increase as a result of the extra work placed on the heart in pushing the blood to the extremities. However, this does not necessarily mean that you are improving your aerobic training, as the increase in the heart rate has no direct correlation to the increase in oxygen usage under these circumstances. Bear this in mind when using arm movements. The 30-minute step programme included in this section does not include arm movements.

Tips for Wise Use of Arms

✦ Use arms mainly for balance and variety. If your arms tire or if you feel strained, drop the arm movements out completely and let the hands sit on the hips. The majority of aerobic work comes from the leg movement so make sure you master the footwork before you add any arm movements.

Hand-held Weights

Research has shown that there is very little benefit from working with hand or wrist weights of less than two pounds. Using heavier weights than this is not advisable while stepping as it can lead to overuse injury, joint strain and also compromise technique quite severely. We recommend that you leave weights out of this programme. If you are keen to work with weights, use them statically, i.e. not while stepping, but when standing still, and at the end of the stepping section.

Use Weights Wisely

✦ Use weights for a specific strength training session only if you have been taught the correct technique for each resistance move.

✦ Don't use weights while stepping, but use them after the stepping section.

Music Speed

Step Reebok is performed most safely at music speeds of between 118 and 122 beats per minute. Using music faster than this means you will not be able to complete the moves properly, and you will increase the risk of injury or tripping. Using music slower than this will make the moves arduous and, for many people, will not raise the training level. Music specifically designed to accompany the Step Reebok programme can be obtained from Muscle Mixes Music (see page 159).

Platform Height

Adjusting the height of your platform to a level that you can easily cope with according to your fitness level and the length of your legs is the most effective way of increasing or decreasing the intensity of the workout. But don't increase too soon or too high, as again this will only impede your progress.

Tips for Safe Platform Heights

✦ Don't increase the platform height until you feel comfortable.

✦ Only increase it by a maximum of two inches at a time, and reduce it again if it feels too difficult to sustain.

✦ Only increase the height for a few moves at a time and build up so you get used to the new height gradually.

✦ Don't be afraid to decrease the platform height and move down a level on the days when you feel less energetic.

✦ Don't increase the platform height beyond the level at which your legs can cope. Untrained long legs will still need to build up gradually until they can cope with the higher levels.

✦ Do not use a platform height that causes the knee to bend beyond 90 degrees when you are stepping on to the platform.

Jumps and Hops

Jumps or hops (otherwise known as propulsions) *increase the intensity quite considerably* and are considered *very* advanced moves. Don't attempt these until you are comfortable. Then learn how to 'power' step properly with a trained instructor.

Duration and Frequency

Gradually increasing the length of time spent stepping or the number of times a week, but keeping to the same intensity level, will show improvements in your fitness and skill level. However when starting out it's better to do a short workout more frequently than attempting to do too much too soon.

The Step Reebok® Platform

There are five extremely important aspects to look for when selecting a step platform for home use. The Step Reebok® platform offers all the following features:

1. Adjustability: Ideally, a platform should be adjustable so that you can change the height to suit your leg length, progress or energy level on any chosen day. For most people, the preferred height for getting the best from the exercise without increasing the risk of injury is approximately eight inches.

2. Stability: The platform should feel completely stable as you place first one foot and then the other foot on it. Test the platform before purchasing, and step up and down on it several times to ensure it does not budge under you.

3. Traction: The top surface of the platform should have sufficient traction to prevent the feet from slipping across it, but not so much traction that it 'catches' your shoes as you try to step on or off.

4. Pliability: A well-designed platform will 'give' a little under your body weight. This may not be perceptible to the naked eye, but it is important for preventing injury from too much impact. As a rule of thumb, most plastic-type materials have a certain amount of 'give'. Avoid wood, metal or solid platforms.

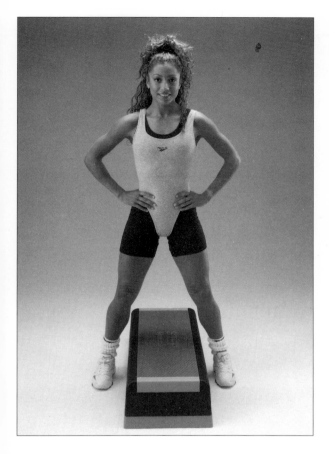

5. Size: One of the most important aspects to look out for is the width of the platform, especially if you don't have particularly long legs. A platform that is too wide is likely to make straddle moves very uncomfortable, but it can also cause you to trip as you struggle to get across it. Always check that you can straddle the platform comfortably before purchasing.

Check the platform is not too wide for you to straddle comfortably.

Step Reebok Terminology and Technique

Posture and Technique Tips

It is important to step with the correct posture. Check your stepping posture and technique as follows:

✦ Always stand straight before stepping, shoulders back and down, chest up.

✦ Stand close to the platform and lean from the ankle not from the hip as you step up.

✦ Pull up out of the hips once on the platform and don't sink down into the hips as you step off, but stand tall.

✦ Don't *bounce* or *funk* on the platform.

✦ *Never* step or jump forward off the platform.

✦ Check that your knees and toes are in alignment.

✦ Don't step on to a platform that is too high for your leg length or strength. The knee should always be lower than the hip when stepping up or down.

✦ Don't let the heels hang off the back of the platform. People with big feet may need to let the toes hang off slightly.

✦ Ensure the foot is flat on the platform and land on the whole foot, not just on the toes.

✦ Land close to the platform when stepping off, and always put the heels down unless doing a lunge or toe touch.

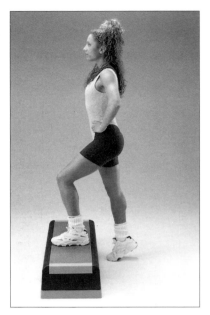

Stand straight, leaning from the ankle, and stand close to the platform. Ensure the foot is always flat on the platform, and land with the whole foot, not just the toes.

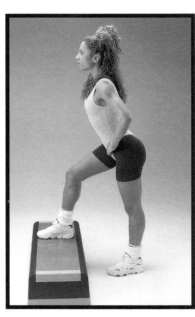

Don't lean from the waist or let your buttocks stick out.

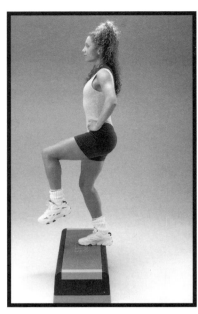

Don't sink into the hips, and don't let the toes or heel hang off the platform.

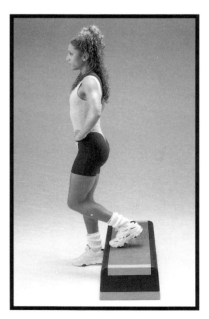

Never step forward off the platform.

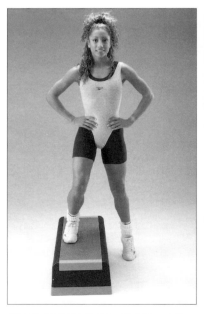

Check that the knees and toes are aligned.

Finding Your Way Around the Platform

Orientation

Step patterns can start from different positions as follows:

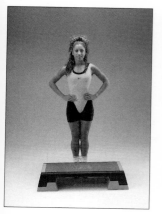
From the front.

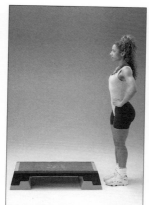
From the end (facing side).

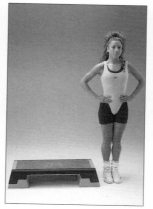
From the end (facing front).

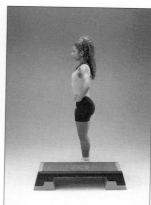
From the side.

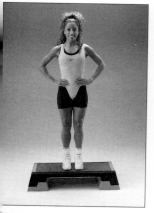
From the top (facing front).

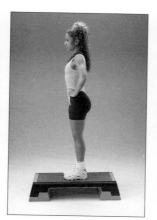
From the top (facing side).

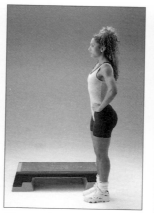
From the corner.

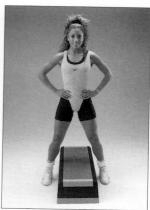
From astride.

The Step Cycle

The step cycle is usually in a count of four. The lead leg is the leg with which you start the cycle. For instance, the Basic Step with the right leg leading is right leg up, left leg up, right leg down, left leg down. You can continue like this and start the next cycle on the same lead leg (single lead move), or you can change lead legs by adding a tap change. To add a tap change, as you bring the leg down you tap the foot to the floor and then bring it straight up on to the platform again. Therefore, the Basic Step with alternating lead leg is right leg up, left leg up, right leg down, left foot comes down to tap the floor (tap change) and goes straight up again to begin the next cycle.

With some moves you use the same lead leg for each cycle, and with moves such as knee lifts you alternate lead legs.

The Core Moves

Learn the core moves first, starting with the Basic Step. Once you are comfortable with the Basic Step, work your way through the rest of the core moves. Practise each one until you feel confident before moving on to the next. When you have mastered them all you will then be ready for the 30-minute workout.

Before you start, check that the platform is stable and on a flat surface, sitting properly on its blocks.

1. The Basic Step ▼

This step is the foundation of the whole programme, and all the other steps are based on this four-count cycle. It is used for warming up, orientation and balance, so familiarize yourself with it before moving on to the other core moves.

Stand close to the platform and, remembering your correct posture and technique, step up on to the platform with the right leg, up with the left leg, down right, down left. Repeat 8 times, then stop and change the lead leg so that you start the cycle with the left leg first.

Caution: Check posture and ankle lean.

Start Positions: From the front, from the end, from the top.

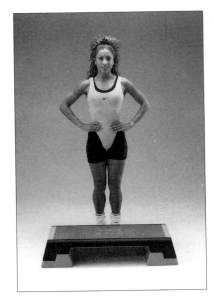
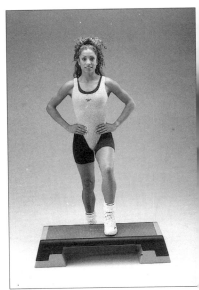

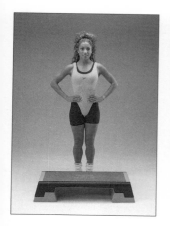 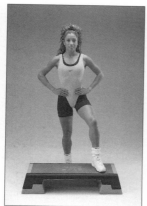 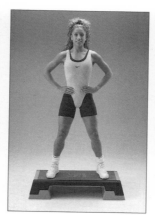 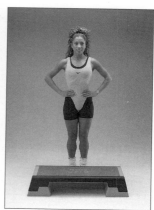

2. The V Step ▲

As the Basic Step, but when you step up take the feet out to each corner of the platform and bring them back together as you step back on the floor.

Caution: Keep stepping close to the platform. Don't lean back. Check that your knees stay in line with your toes.

Start Positions: From the front only.

Safety Tip

✦ **To avoid overuse injury or muscle imbalance, limit single lead step cycles to a maximum of one minute or 30 cycles before changing the lead leg so that both legs are worked equally.**

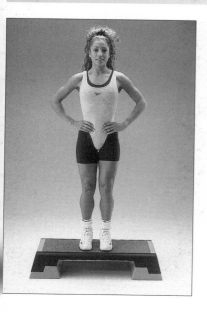 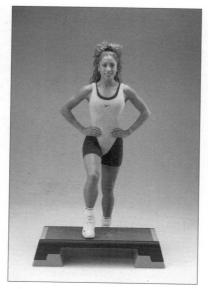 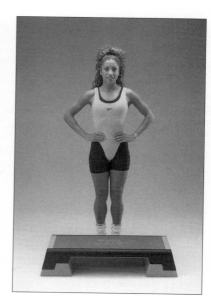

3. Tap Up Tap Down ▶

Step up right, tap the left toe on top of the platform, step down left, tap the right toe on the floor. Step up right again and continue like this.

Start Positions: From the front, from the end, from the corner, from the side, from the top (tap down, tap up).

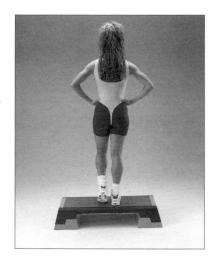 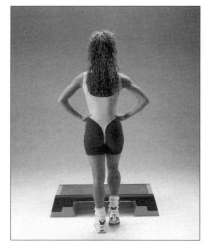

4. Straddle Down ▶

Start on top of the platform, facing one end. Step down right, step down left, step up right, step up left.

Start Positions: From the top only.

To change lead legs, tap on top of the platform.

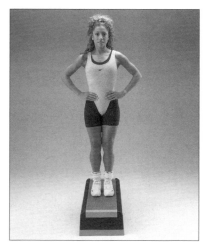 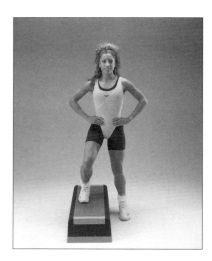

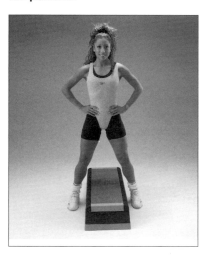 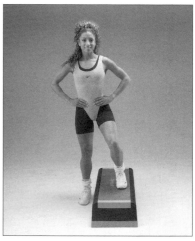 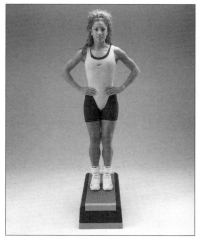

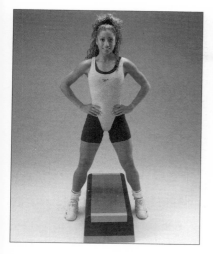
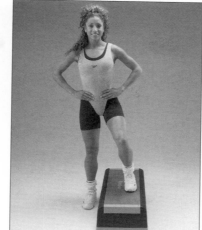
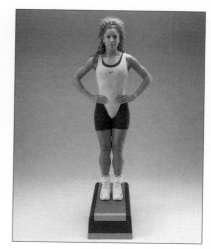
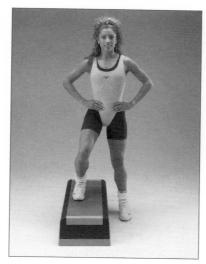
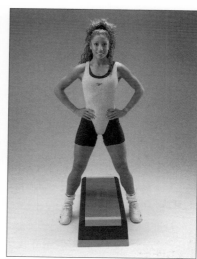

5. Straddle Up

Start astride the platform. Step up right, step up left, down right, down left.

Caution: Ensure your knees are always in line with your toes and not rolling in. Land with the whole foot when stepping on to the platform or back down to the floor. If the platform is too wide for your leg length, omit this step.

Start Positions: From astride only.

To change lead legs, tap on the floor.

6. Leg Lifts

These include knee lifts, hamstring curls, leg lifts front or leg lifts side. Moves which involve lifting the legs will increase the intensity and will help improve balance, coordination and agility. The stepping pattern is the same in all.

Caution: Check posture. Leg lifts tend to throw the weight away from the raising leg. Be sure to correct your posture — don't lean away from the leg or arch your spine. Keep the leg movements low and strong. Knee lifts should be no higher than hip level, and leg lifts no higher than mid-calf level.

Start Positions: From the front, from astride, from the end, from the side.

Knee Lift ▶

Step up right, lift the left knee, step down left, step down right (4 counts). Step up left, lift the right knee, step down right, step down left (8 counts).

Leg Lift Side ▼

As above but replace the knee lift with a leg lift to the side.

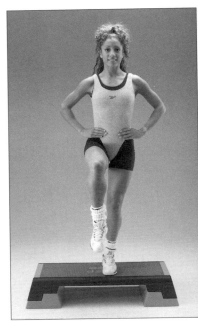

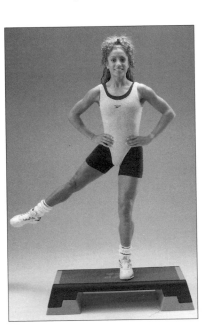

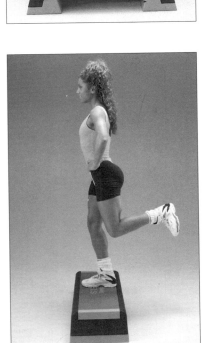

Hamstring Curl ◀

As above but replace the knee lift with a hamstring curl.

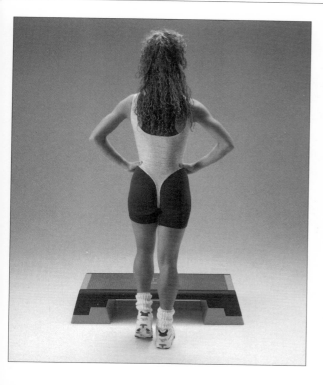

7. Alternating Tap Down ◄

Step up right, step up left, step down right, tap down left (4 counts). Step up left, up right, down left, tap down right (8 counts).

Caution: Check posture and knee alignment.

Start Positions: From the front, from astride, from the end.

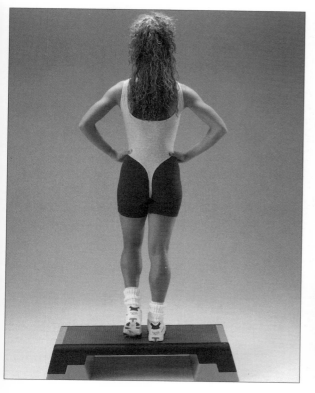

8. Alternating Tap Up ◄

As Tap Down but start on top and reverse the sequence. Step down right, step down left, step up right, tap up left (4 counts). Step down left, step down right, step up left, tap up right (8 counts).

Caution: Check posture and knee alignment.

Start Positions: From the front, from astride, from the end.

Alternating Tap Down and Alternating Tap Up can be used as 'breather' steps or for changing legs, or as preparation for turn steps (as you tap down gradually turn to the side) or lift steps (replace tap up with a lift step).

9. Over the Top

This is used as a travelling step and improves agility, balance and coordination.

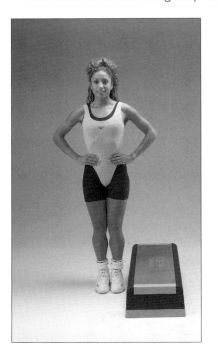
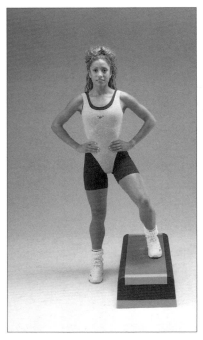
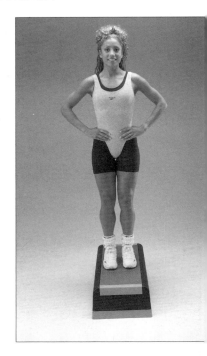

Stand sideways on to the platform. Step up with the leg closest to the platform, step up with the other leg so you are standing on top facing the end, step down on the other side (4 counts). Repeat to return to the start position (8 counts).

Caution: Check knee alignment – don't let the knees roll in as you step up. Limit to a maximum of 8 repetitions to avoid strain on the knees.

Start Positions: From the side only.

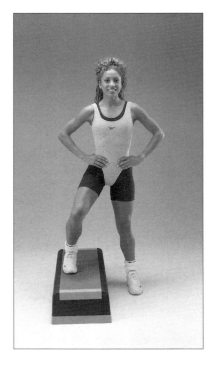
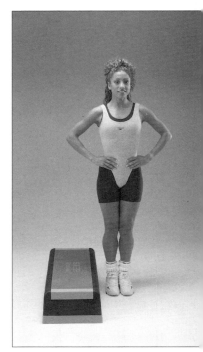

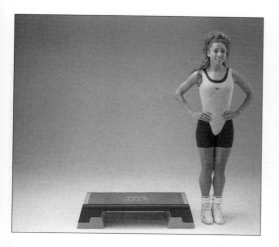
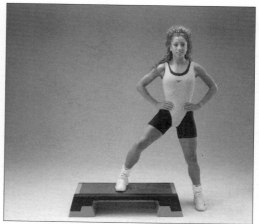

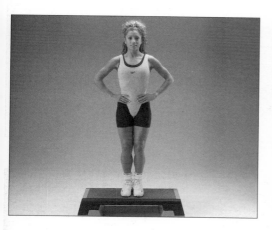
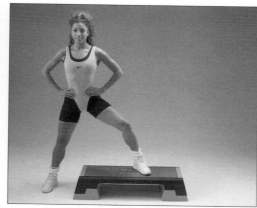

10. Across the Top

Stand at one end of the platform facing the front of the room. Step up with the leg closest to the platform as far into the platform as you can comfortably reach, step up with the other leg, step down off the other end (4 counts). Repeat to return to the start position (8 counts).

Caution: Check that the knees remain aligned. Add a little hop to get you across the top if it helps. As this is an advanced move, limit to one minute (approximately 4 cycles) to prevent overloading the knees, and ensure the platform height is adjusted appropriately for your needs.

Alternatively, replace with the following move.

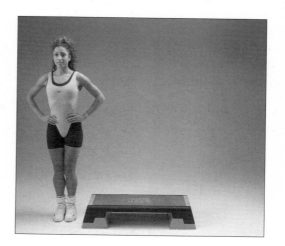

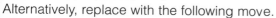

Alternative move to Across the Top

Start at one end of the platform as before and take two steps along the floor to the opposite end of the platform. Repeat, taking two steps to come back to your start position.

Start Positions: From the end only.

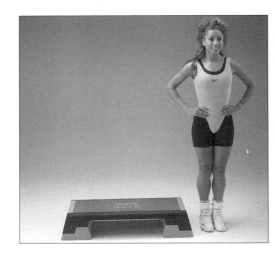

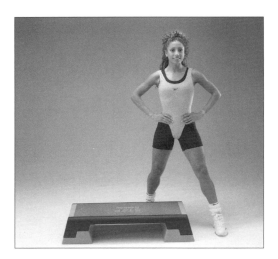

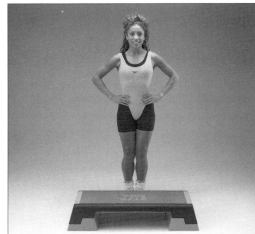

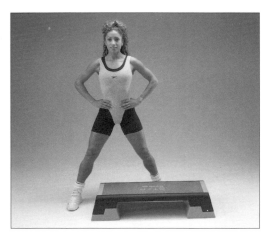

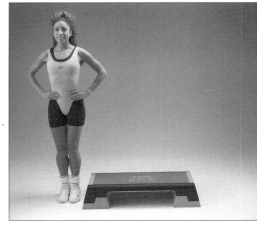

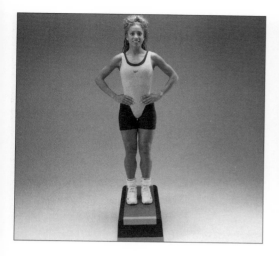
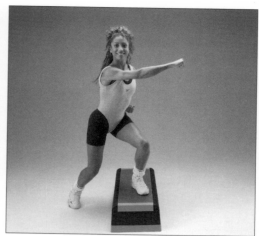
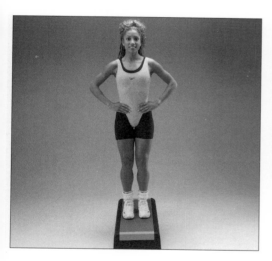
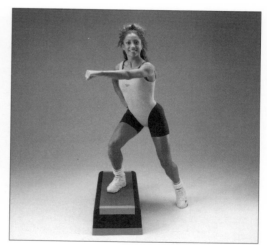

11. Lunges

These are used to add variety and as preparation for propulsions (jumps). They also help improve flexibility, coordination and balance.

Start from the top facing the end. Touch the toe (but *not* the heel) down to the floor, bring the foot back on to the platform (4 counts) and touch the other toe down (8 counts). The slow version takes 4 counts each leg, and the fast version takes 2 counts each leg.

Caution: Check knee alignment – don't let the knees roll in and don't put the full weight on the lowering toe. As these are advanced moves limit to one minute to avoid strain on the knees. Keep your posture upright and don't stick your buttocks out.

Start Positions: From the top only.

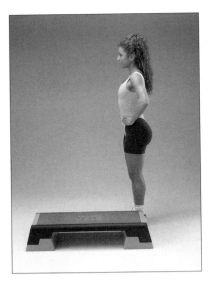
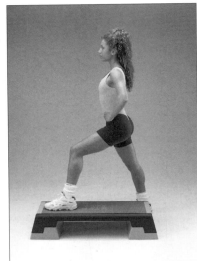
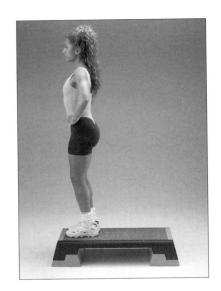

12. The A Step

Stand at the corner of the platform, facing the side of the room, with your right leg nearest the platform. Step up and forward with the right leg, towards the opposite end of the platform. Step up with the left, step back with the right leg to the floor at the opposite corner from where you started. Bring the left leg back and tap the toe to the floor ready to repeat with the left leg leading (4 counts). Repeat with the left leg to complete the cycle and take you back to your original start position (8 counts).

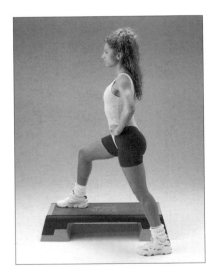
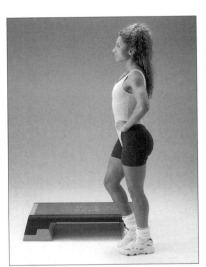

Caution: Check that the knees stay aligned and pay extra attention when stepping backward.

Start Positions: From the corner, from the side, from the front.

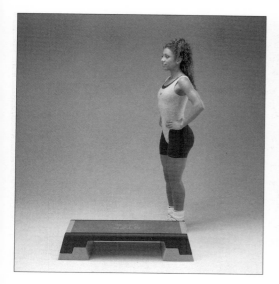
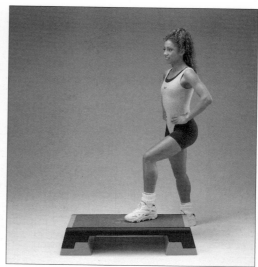
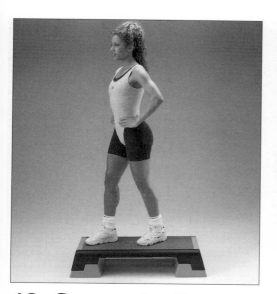
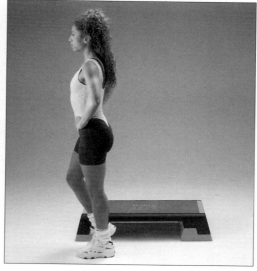

13. Corner to Corner

Stand at the corner of the platform, with your right leg closest to it and face the opposite end. Step up with the right leg (heading for the diagonally opposite corner), step up with the left, step off with the right leg to the floor at the corner, step off with the left leg (4 counts).Walk back to the end of the platform for 4 counts. You are now on the opposite side of the platform to your start position. Repeat the whole sequence to return to your original start position (6 counts).

Caution: Check knee alignment.

Start Positions: From the corner only.

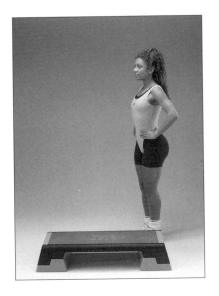
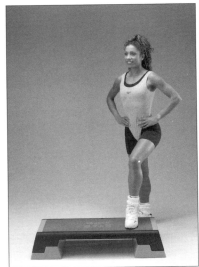
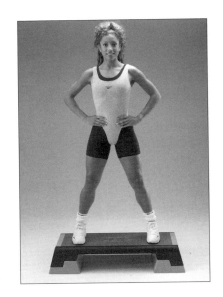

14. Turn Step

Stand sideways on at the right-hand side corner of the platform and face the opposite end. Step up with the right leg to the right end of the platform, step up with the left to the other end of the platform, step off with the right leg to the opposite end (but still to the same side of the platform), step off with the left. You should now be facing the place from where you started (4 counts). Step up with the left and repeat the sequence to return to your original start position (8 counts).

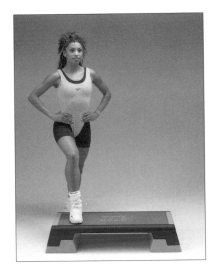
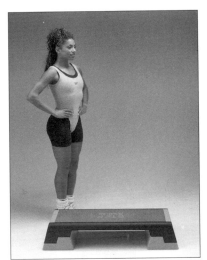

Caution: Check knee alignment – make sure your knees are over your toes and that they don't twist as you turn. If you have problems with dizziness limit turns to 4 repetitions of the full cycle. Begin the first step by turning the leg out from the hip, not the knee.

Start Positions: From the corner only.

Practice Makes Perfect

Practise the core moves with or without music until you can perform each one comfortably. (This is a good time to have your technique checked by an approved Reebok instructor or by going along to a Step Reebok® class.)

Once you have mastered the core moves, you can attempt the 30-minute workout. Use the warm-up and cool-down sections from the Basic Workout. Remember to keep the moves slow and controlled, and aim for quality of movement rather than quantity.

The Step Reebok® Workout

Format

	Approximate time
Warm-up and stretch	5 minutes
Orientation	2 minutes
Aerobics routines	20 minutes
Cool-down and stretch	5 minutes

The aerobics section is divided into three routines. Each routine takes approximately one minute. Always start and finish with Routine 1 to give yourself a gentle start and wind-down to the aerobics section.

For 20 minutes of aerobic work:

Repeat Routine 1 four times (twice starting right lead leg, twice starting left lead leg).

Repeat Routine 2 four times (twice on each lead leg).

Repeat Routine 3 four times (twice on each lead leg).

Repeat Routine 2 four times (twice on each lead leg).

Repeat Routine 1 four times (twice on each lead leg).

For a less strenuous aerobics section:

Repeat Routines 2 and 3 twice only.

Complete beginners should always do this version and use the lower end of the music speed range.

For extra challenge:

Do further repetitions of each routine, making sure you do an equal number of repetitions on each lead leg.

Warm-up and Stretch

Music speed: 125–135 bpm

Use the warm-up and stretch from the Basic Workout, then spend a couple of minutes on orientation before you move on to the aerobics routines.

Orientation

+ Stand in front of the platform and march on the floor for 16 counts.
+ Step up and down, doing the Basic Step very slowly and taking 2 counts for each step (8 counts in all). Repeat once more.
+ Take 16 counts to walk all the way around the platform in a clockwise direction.
+ March on the spot for 16 counts.
+ Walk around the platform in the opposite direction and take 16 counts.
+ Stand on the platform and shuffle to one end for 4 counts, back to the middle for 4, then to the other end for 4 and back to the middle for 4.
+ Step back off the platform and walk around it for 8 counts anticlockwise, then 8 counts clockwise.

Aerobics Routines

Music speed: 118–120 bpm

Now that you are familiar with all the moves, you are ready to put them together. Have a practice run first with each of these routines. Don't move on to the next routine until you are comfortable with the previous one.

The number of times you repeat a step is marked on the left and the total number of counts on the right. Each footfall or leg move has a count (or music beat) of its own, so count it out as you mark it through. Remember each routine takes approximately one minute, so repeat as indicated for 20 minutes of aerobic work. Each time you repeat a routine, start on a different lead leg.

Remember to take your pulse or perceived exertion at the end of each routine.

Note: Alt = alternating lead leg, R = right lead leg, L = left lead leg.

Routine 1

Approximate time: 1 minute

Stand at the front of the platform, and start with the right leg.

No. of reps	Core move	Total counts
4	**Basic Step** R (tap change on count 16, ready to step L)	16
4	**Basic Step** L	16
4	**Alt Tap Up** (step L, tap up R 1st) (tap down R on count 16, ready to step R)	16
4	**Basic Step** R	16
4	**Alt Knee Lift** (step up R, lift L knee 1st) (tap down L on count 16, ready to step L)	16
4	**Basic Step** L	16
4	**Alt Leg Lift Side** (step L, lift R leg 1st) (tap down R on count 16, ready to step R)	16
4	**Basic Step** R	16
4	**Alt Hamstring Curl** (step R, lift L leg 1st) (tap down L on count 16, ready to step L)	16
	Basic Step L	16

Repeat the whole routine, starting with the left leg.

For the practice run: Repeat until you get it right. Ensure you change the lead leg each time.

For the 20-minute aerobics workout: Repeat 4 times in all, twice on each lead leg (4 minutes).

Safety Tip : Never stay on the same lead leg for more than one minute.

Routine 2

Approximate time: 1 minute

Stand in front of the platform and start with the right leg.

No. of reps	Core move	Total counts
2	**Basic Step** L (tap change on count 8, ready to step R)	8
4	**Basic Step** R	8
4	**Alt Tap Down** (step R, tap L 1st) (finish sideways on, R leg nearest the platform)	16
4	**Turn Step** (R 1st)	16
4	**Over the Top** (R 1st)	16
4	**A Step** (R 1st)	16
2	**Corner to Corner** (R 1st) (walk back to start position each time)	16
3	**Turn Step** (R 1st) (you are now facing the other way)	12
1	**Tap Up** R, **Tap Down** L	4
4	**Over the Top** (L 1st)	16
4	**A Step** (L 1st)	16
2	**Corner to Corner** (L 1st) (walk back to start position each time)	16
3	**Turn Step** (L 1st) (you are now facing the original way)	12
3	**Tap Up** R, **Tap Down** L	12
2	**Step up** R **and march on top**	8

Repeat the whole routine starting with the left leg.

For the practice run: Repeat until you feel confident with the sequence of moves. Remember to change the lead leg each time.

For the 20-minute aerobics workout: Repeat 4 times in all, twice on each lead leg, (4 minutes).

Routine 3

Approximate time: 1 minute
Start on top, with the right leg leading.

No. of reps	Core move	Total counts
4	**Straddle Down** R (on last straddle tap L on top, ready to step L)	16
4	**Straddle Down** L	16
8	**Lunges** (R 1st, 4 counts each leg) (rhythm slows down)	32
1	**Step backward off the end** (R 1st) (back to speed for the marching)	4
4	**March** R **on the spot**, from the end	4
4	**Basic Step** R, from the end	16
2	**Alt Leg Lift Side**, from the end (step R, lift L 1st)	8
8	**March** R, turning sideways on to the platform (tap change on count 8, ready to march L)	8
8	**March** L **on the spot**	8
1	**Across the Top** L **to the other end**	4
4	**March** R **on the spot**	4
1	**Across the Top** R	4
4	**March** L **on the spot**	4
1	**March** L **around the platform** (anticlockwise) (finish at the front start position)	16
16	**Step up** L **and march on top,** turning sideways (you are ready to start the routine again on the other leg)	16

For the practice run: Repeat until the sequence flows comfortably. Remember to change the lead leg each time.

For the 20-minute aerobics workout: Repeat 4 times in all, twice on each lead leg (4 minutes), then continue as follows:

Repeat Routine 2 four times, twice on each lead leg (4 minutes).

Repeat Routine 1 four times, twice on each lead leg (4 minutes).

Cool-down and Stretch

Music speed: 90–100 bpm
Never stop suddenly – always slow down gradually.

No. of reps

8	**Basic Step** R, very slow, taking 8 counts each
8	**March** R **on the top**
8	**March** R **on the floor**
16	**Walk** R **around the platform**
16	**Walk** L **around the platform**
8	**March** L **on the spot**

For the 30-minute workout, turn to page 72 for the final stretch. If you wish to add a strengthening session, turn to page 66 and follow the cool-down instructions before doing any strengthening work. Always finish with the final stretch.

Congratulations! You have now completed the Step Reebok programme.

Slide Reebok

Slide Reebok™ is the most skill-oriented of all the Reebok University training programmes, so don't be surprised if it takes you a little longer than you expect to master the art of sliding. The more time you spend on getting the technique right, the more fun you'll have later with the work-out.

What Is Slide Reebok?

Slide Reebok™ training is technically termed 'lateral movement training'. This is because it involves sideways movements, and therefore trains the muscles used in these movements. Most of our daily activities are in a backward/forward or up/down direction, as are most sports activities or forms of fitness training. Therefore, the muscles and connective tissue in the sides of the legs, both outer and inner, tend to be underused.

However, some sports require sudden lateral actions. So, training the inner and outer legs is particularly useful for sports people who use sideways-type moves, for example the soccer player passing the ball or the tennis player lunging to the side. Slide training can help improve strength and agility in this area.

What Does It Involve?

Very simply, it involves sliding from side to side across a specially designed mat with safety bumpers at each end. Simple as that sounds, a fair amount of skill is required, but this can be quickly learned, and the body will soon adapt (even if the mind takes a little longer!).

Who Should Do It?

Any reasonably fit and healthy adult with some exercise experience and good motor skills will be able to learn the skills involved. Slide Reebok can be adapted to suit different levels of ability but, like any exercise programme, it needs to be undertaken *gradually*.

What Will It Do For Me?

Slide Reebok is an excellent way of toning up the lower body, particularly those flabby inner thighs. It is also a good method of aerobic training, and can improve balance, agility and lower body strength.

Slide Reebok: The Benefits

+ A low-impact activity.
+ A useful aid to weight loss.
+ Great for toning legs and buttocks.
+ Forms a good aerobic workout.
+ Complements sports training.
+ Can be used with or without music.
+ Can be used at home or in a class.
+ Improves agility and balance.

While Slide Reebok can be a useful aid to weight loss (see page 157 for approximate energy expenditure), it is not advisable to use it as your sole exercise activity, as this could lead to overtraining certain muscle groups and increased risk of injury. Because the Slide Reebok programme uses the generally underused inner thigh muscles (adductors), you may at first experience a little muscle soreness in this area. Even seasoned exercisers or sports people may feel sore after their first few attempts at sliding because their regular activity does not greatly involve these muscles. The soreness should pass within two to seven days, but in the meantime you can carry out an alternative activity that doesn't focus on this muscle area.

Where to Start

The Slide Reebok programme has specific recommendations for starting out. Bearing in mind that sliding does to a certain extent have a spot-training effect on vulnerable muscle tissue, we suggest you err strongly on the side of caution. Select your moves from the chart on page 124. To avoid overtraining as you start out consider the following guidelines.

Entry Level 1

This is the start point for *everyone*. Even if you are 'aerobically' fit you will still need time to acclimatize. Limit the on-board activity to between five and ten minutes for the first four to five sessions. The aim is to master the Basic Slide move. Only when you can manoeuvre back and forth across the board quite easily should you move on to the next entry level.

Entry Level 2

The aim here is to become proficient in all of the low- and mid-intensity core moves (see page 124). Don't at this stage attempt to link the different moves together, but just aim to master the correct alignment and posture. Limit the on-board activity to between five and ten minutes. Move on to Level 3 only when you are confident with all of these moves and can perform eight consecutive slides of each move.

Entry Level 3

Now aim to link together in a continuous movement the core moves you learned in Level 2. Do not do more than eight consecutive slides of any one move, and intersperse them with the Basic Slide. Limit the on-board activity to between 10 and 20 minutes.

Entry Level 4

Once you can link the low- and mid-intensity core moves proficiently, try adding the high-intensity core moves, but, again, do not attempt more than eight consecutive slides of any one move. Intersperse them with the Basic Slide to maintain the balance of the workload. Limit the on-board activity to 20 minutes, and ensure you stay within your training heart rate zone.

How Often to Practise

Until you have completed all levels it is recommended that you slide just once a week. Spend at least five sessions at Level 1, and at least three sessions at the other levels. When you arrive at Level 4, you can build up gradually to three times a week. Use the entry level guidelines to put together your own workout. Once you are proficient at Level 4 you can then attempt the 30-minute workout (see page 134), and your weekly schedule could look something like this.

Suggested Weekly Schedule

Monday	Slide Reebok	30 minutes	30-minute workout
Tuesday	Walk Reebok	30 minutes	4 mph
Wednesday	Rest		
Thursday	Swimming	30 minutes	Splash about
Friday	Slide Reebok	30 minutes	30-minute workout
Saturday	Aqua aerobics	60 minutes	Beginners
Sunday	Rest		

The Four Phases of the Programme

1. **Entry: complete all four entry levels.**
2. **Introductory: ready to attempt the 30-minute workout.**
3. **Intermediate: competent at the workout.**
4. **Advanced: experienced at the workout.**

Slide Reebok Terminology and Technique

Before you learn to slide you need to familiarize yourself with the board itself, the safety factors and technique, plus the terms used to describe the different aspects of sliding.

The Slide Reebok Board

Although it looks like a heavy duty mat, the slide is actually referred to as a board. This is because the Norwegian skiers and skaters who developed this training system some 100 years ago used wooden boards. Based on the original Norwegian concept, the Slide Reebok board has been designed with safety and effectiveness in mind.

The board is lightweight, durable and easily portable. It rolls up for storage, and easily rolls out flat for use. There are end ramps at each end to help with the 'push off' and 'recovery' phases of the Basic Slide. The end ramps are angled to allow for the natural angle of the foot as well as to slow down the move. Each ramp has a small 90-degree bumper that acts as a 'brake' to ensure the slider does not overshoot the ramp.

The sliding surface is designed to be 'slick' for gliding yet have sufficient friction to aid balance and create resistance in order to work the leg muscles.

Safety Precautions

+ Always make sure the board lies flat with the Reebok logo facing you so that you can read it. This enables the end ramps to serve their purpose.
+ Before using the board always make sure the strap is not underneath it.
+ Never slide backward on the board.
+ Never jump, jive or funk on the board.
+ Don't allow children on to the board without adult supervision.
+ Never polish or wet the sliding surface of the board.
+ Never use weights, bands or equipment while sliding on the board.
+ Always warm up before using the board.
+ Always put on your Slide Reebok socks before you get on to the board.
+ Only use the board for the activity it was designed for – sliding.

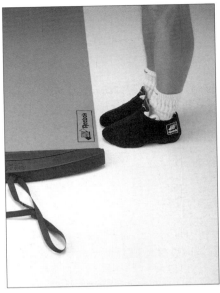

Make sure the Reebok logo is facing you.

Sliding Technique

Start Positions

There are three start positions: from the front, from the end, and from the centre. Each move will start or finish at one of these points, but the front is the one that is most frequently used.

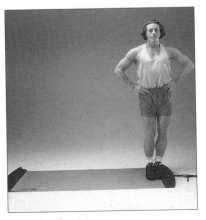

From the front.

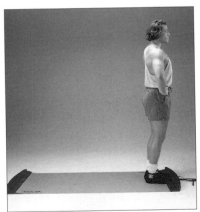

From the end.

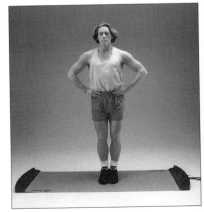

From the centre.

Posture

There are two stances: the *upright stance*, which is used for beginners, or the more advanced *athletic ready stance*.

Upright Stance

Stay upright, keeping the chest and the chin up (don't look at the board) and the shoulders, hips and knees in alignment. Knees should always be slightly bent when sliding, and in line with the toes.

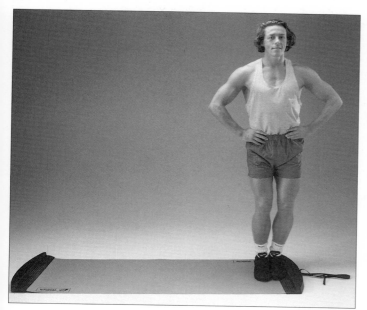

Correct posture upright stance (front view).

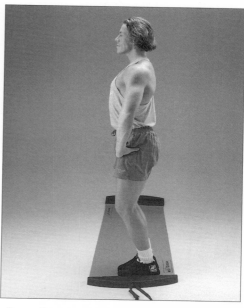

Correct posture upright stance (side view).

Athletic Ready Stance

Keep the posture aligned and push the buttocks back as if going into a squat. Don't lean forward from the waist. Instead, it should feel as if you were about to sit down. To begin with, keep your hands on your thighs or behind your back. Keep your weight evenly distributed between your feet to help keep your balance.

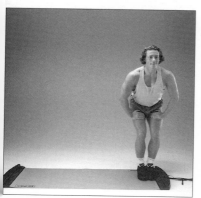

Correct posture athletic ready stance (front view).

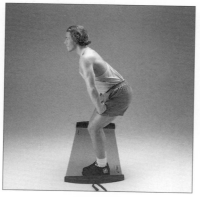

Correct posture athletic ready stance (side view).

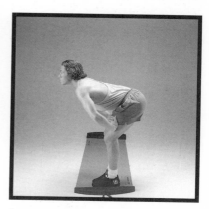

Incorrect posture (side view).

Legs

The leg nearest the ramp is called the *trail leg* and the leg nearest the direction in which you are going to slide is the *lead leg*. The trail leg pushes off, then drags during the glide. The lead leg contacts the ramp first, followed by the trail leg. After recovery, the trail leg becomes the lead leg.

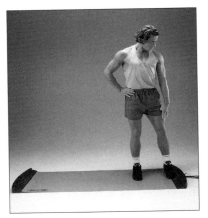

Trail leg.

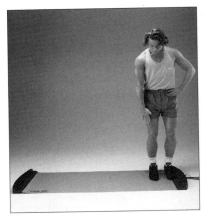

Lead leg.

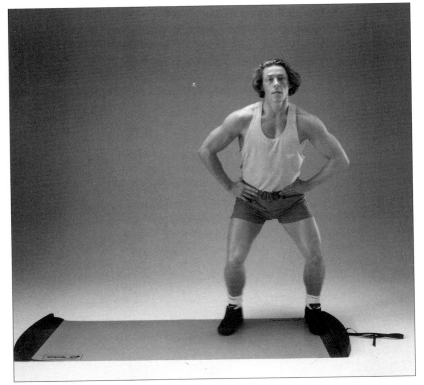

The Sliding Process

The Basic Slide breaks down into three phases: the *push off*, the *glide* and the *recovery*.

Push Off

Stand with both feet together, with the trail leg as close to the 90-degree bumper as possible. Push off by pressing down into the ramp with the trail leg.

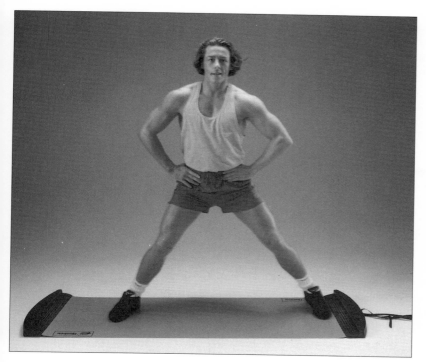

Glide

Stay upright, with head and shoulders facing forward (don't look at the board). You need to keep the legs wide apart – much wider than at first feels comfortable. The weight should be evenly distributed between both legs, and both feet should be absolutely flat against the surface of the slide. At this point, increase the resistance and concentrate on leaving the trail leg as far away from you as possible, but at the same time push it down on to the slide so that it feels as if it is dragging behind you. This 'dragging' helps you to slow down by acting as a type of break. The wider the legs, the more you will keep your balance.

Recovery

Aim to land right up on the ramp. Your posture should remain upright, with knees still bent and feet flat. The trail leg should not come in until the very last second. Make sure you have landed on the ramp and are stable before pushing off again.

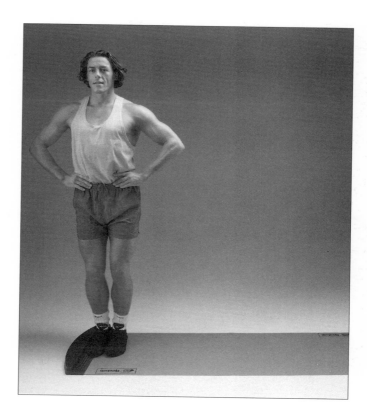

Warm-up and Stretch

Always warm up off the board. Be sure to warm up even if you are just trying out the board for the first time. Use the warm-up and stretch from the Basic Workout, but add the following before starting the slide section:

Lunges

Do 8 to alternate sides, then hold the last one for 30 seconds to stretch out the inner thigh (see page 64). Do 8 more lunges, then hold to the other side for 30 seconds.

Side leg raises

Do 8 to alternate sides. After the last raise, cross the leg in front and hold for 30 seconds to stretch out the outer thigh (see page 63). Repeat, and hold on the other leg.

Stepping on to the Slide

Sit down to put on your Slide Reebok™ socks. When the socks are on stand up and test the board for slipperiness with one foot only (just like you would test the bath water). Now step on to the ramp to practise your first slide. Always start and finish each move tidily and end back up on the ramp as close to the 90-degree bumper as possible. The ramp is etched so that it acts as a stabilizer and prevents you from slipping over when balancing on one leg.

Don't aim to get all the way across first time. Do the 'inch worm', which allows you to progress gradually.

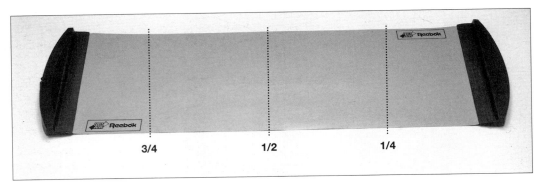

3/4   1/2   1/4

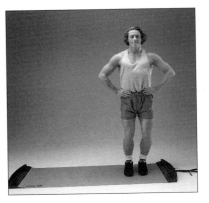
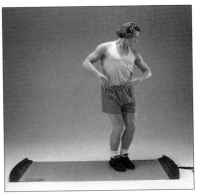

The Inch Worm

Stand at one end of the board, with feet together and the trail leg up against the 90-degree bumper. Push off with the trail leg and aim only for a quarter of the way across. Inch your way back to the ramp. Repeat twice.

Inch your way back.

Now push off and aim for halfway across, then inch your way back. Repeat twice.

This time, aim for three-quarters of the way across, then inch your way over to the other end. Repeat from this side.

Repeat until you find yourself sliding all the way across. Now check your posture and your positioning on the ramp.

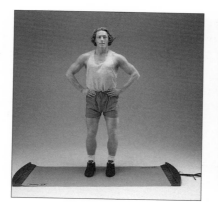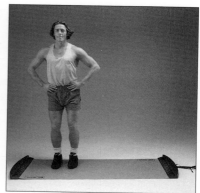

Congratulations, you are now sliding!

Technique Tips

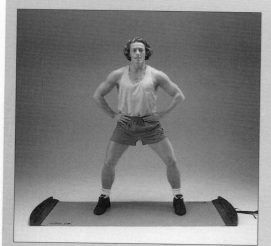

✦ Knees should always be slightly bent, in line with the toes and not rolling in or out.

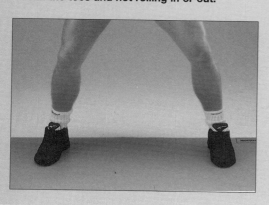

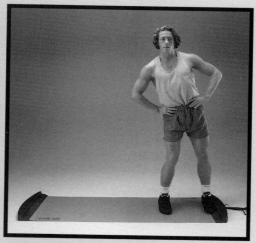

✦ Shoulders should always be square and not leaning in the direction of the slide or forward or backward.

✦ Feet should always be flat on the board surface. Don't let them lift (see left).

✦ Don't have the legs too narrow as you slide or you will topple over.

✦ If it hurts, don't do it! Stop and see a Slide Reebok instructor to find out the cause of the problem.

The Core Moves

There are fifteen core moves in the Slide Reebok programme. Once you have learned these you will be ready to slide and be able to put your own workout together. For the purpose of this programme the core moves are divided into three measures of intensity according to the demands made up on the body. These are as follows:

Entry Level 1	Entry Levels 2 and 3	Entry Level 4
Low Intensity	**Mid Intensity**	**High Intensity**
(Less than 70% MHRR)	*(70–80% MHRR)*	*(Greater than 80% MHRR)*
Basic Slide	Slide Touch Front	Low Profile Slide (in 2 counts)
	Slide Touch Rear	Leg Lift Side
	Knee Lift Front	Slide Lunge Rear
	Knee Lift Across	Cross Country Wide
	Knee Lift Side	Slide Squat
	Hamstring Curl	Slide Lift Double
	Leg Lift Front	Slide Lift Single
	Leg Lift Rear	Squat Pull
	Fencing Slide	Wide Slide
	Reverse Fencing Slide	
	Cross Country Narrow	
	Slide Lunge Side	
	Speed Skate	
	Low Profile Slide (in 4 counts)	

Factors Affecting Intensity

When exercising, remember there are certain factors that affect how hard you are working. Use the pulse rate checks and perceived exertion chart on pages 25–26 to keep a check on your exertion level to ensure you are getting the full benefits without overtraining. If you follow the guidelines in this programme you should be able to stay within your training heart rate zone.

However, there are other factors to be aware of which will influence the intensity of the exercise.

✦ Speed of the slide. Follow the recommended speeds and cadences here. Increasing the speed will increase the intensity, so don't go too fast.

✦ Arm movements (especially overhead). Avoid too many arm movements. Keep your arms on your waist or behind your back, or use as counterbalance.

✦ Types of moves. Follow the guidelines for the entry levels, and keep high-intensity moves to a minimum. Use the low- and mid-intensity moves for most of the workout, using the high-intensity moves to increase the challenge occasionally.

◆ Drag of the trail leg. Dragging the trail leg increases the intensity of the workout. Not dragging means you are more liable to lose your balance and you will also get less of an aerobic effect.

◆ Board surface. Keep it clean but *not* polished. If it is too slippery it will cause balance problems. If it is not slippery enough it will increase the drag effect.

Technique for the Core Moves

1. Basic Slide

The Basic Slide is the foundation of the whole programme and can be used as a breather in between intermediate and advanced moves and to regain balance and posture.

Stand at one end of the board with feet together and the trail leg up against the 90-degree bumper. Push off with the trail leg. Keep your legs wide with your weight evenly distributed and concentrate on leaving your trail leg as far away from you as possible. Land right up on the ramp and only bring your trail leg in at the very last second. Make sure you have landed on the ramp before pushing off again.

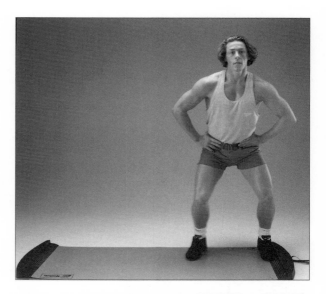

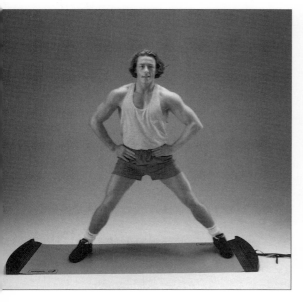

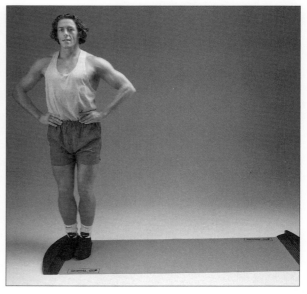

2. Slide Touch Front or Rear ▶

Complete the Basic Slide and make sure you have made solid contact with the end ramp before initiating the toe touch. Lift the trail leg and touch either the end ramp or the edge of the board, in front of or behind your lead leg.

Caution: Be careful not to lean backward or forward as you extend the foot. Keep the posture upright.

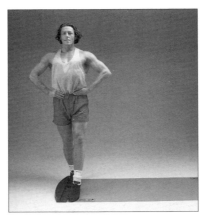

Slide Touch Front.

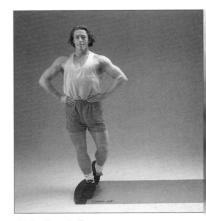

Slide Touch Rear.

3. Knee Lift Front, Side or Across▼

Caution: Remember your posture. Don't lift the knee too high – keep it below hip height – and don't sink into the hips.

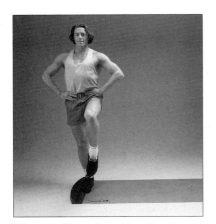

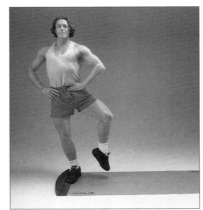

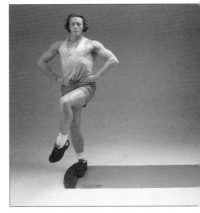

Front: Complete the Basic Slide and lift the knee of the trail leg straight up in front of the body.

Side: Complete the Basic Slide and rotate the trail leg outward as you lift the knee to the side.

Across: Complete the Basic Slide and lift the trail leg, bringing the knee across the body.

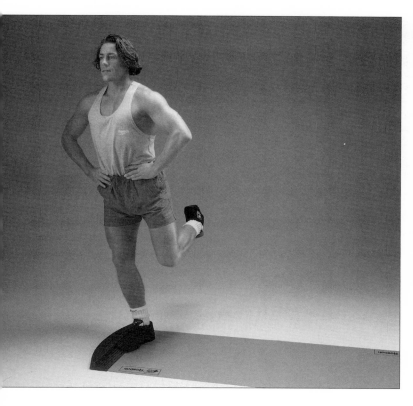

4. Hamstring Curl ◀

Complete the Basic Slide and lift the heel of your trail leg towards your buttocks, using a slow, steady motion.

Caution: Keep the foot at knee height and keep the knees level to maintain good alignment and balance. Don't arch the spine.

5. Leg Lift Front Rear or Side ▶

Complete the Basic Slide, then stabilize the lead leg on the ramp and kick to the front, back or side, keeping the foot at mid-shin height. Don't lean away from the kick or lift the leg too high.

Caution: Ensure the supporting leg stays in alignment.

Note: Leg Lift Side (not illustrated) is a high intensity move, so if you attempt this move proceed with caution.

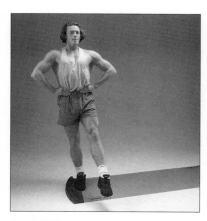

Leg Lift Front.

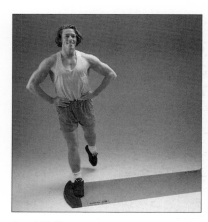

Leg Lift Rear.

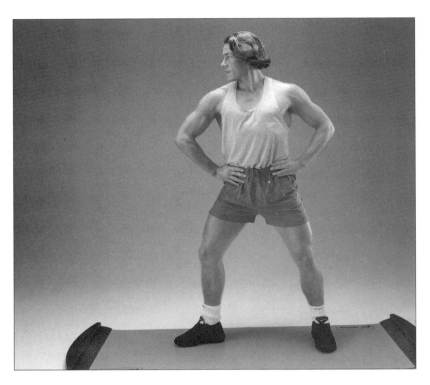

6. Fencing Slide ◄

This is similar to the Basic Slide but as you slide, rotate the lead leg outward so that it 'cuts' through the centre of the board as if you were in a fencing position. Turn the lead foot to the front again as you make contact with the end ramp.

Caution: Ensure the knees and toes are always facing the same direction. Limit the number of repetitions as this is used mainly as a transition move.

7. Reverse Fencing Slide ►

This time, slide with the lead leg in the normal position and rotate the trail leg outward. Maintain the drag, but the work should come more from the hamstrings (back of thighs) than the adductors (inner thighs).

Caution: Take care to keep the knees and toes in alignment. Don't twist the knee against the direction of the body, but let the hips follow the move.

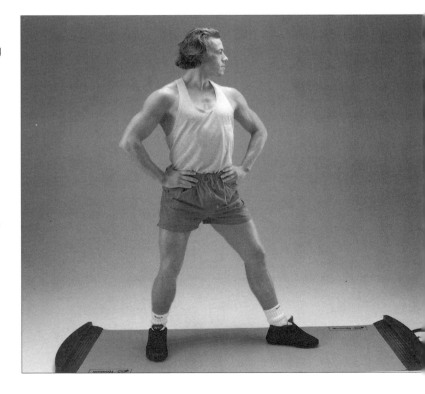

8. Cross Country Narrow and Wide

Narrow: Face the end ramp with both toes on the ramp. Slide one foot backward as far as possible but keep the heel flat, then pull back to the start position and repeat with the other leg. Continue sliding alternate feet backward and forward. Swing the arms in opposition to aid balance if necessary.

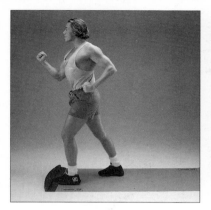 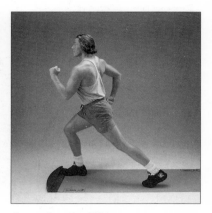

Cross Country Narrow.   **Cross Country Wide.**

Wide: Start from the end position with both toes on the ramp. This time, lunge back with one foot as far as possible, raising the heel, then pull back to the start position and repeat with the other leg.

Caution: Always keep one toe anchored on the ramp. Don't bend the knee beyond the toe or drop the hips below the level of the front knee. Don't hop or bounce, but ensure you slide the feet backward and forward.

9. Slide Lunge Side and Rear

Slide Lunge Side: This can be performed stationary or in combination with the Basic Slide. Complete the Basic Slide and stabilize your lead leg on the end ramp. Push the trail leg back out along the board and pull it in again before beginning the next slide. Keep the foot flat on the board and only go as far as feels comfortable.

Caution: Keep the knees aligned with the toes, and don't let the supporting knee roll in. Bend from the knees not the waist.

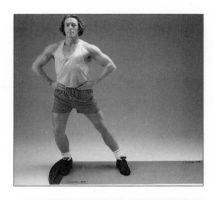

Slide Lunge Rear: This is similar to the Cross Country move, but the focus is on one leg at a time. Start from the end with toes anchored on the ramp. Lunge back with one leg as far as possible, then pull back to the start position and repeat on the same leg for 2, 4, 6 or 8 repetitions (as many as is comfortable). Repeat on the other leg. (This move can also be combined with the Basic Slide or Fencing Slide.)

Caution: Don't let the hips drop below knee level. Be sure to slide the foot backward and forward, and don't hop or bounce. Keep the head at the same height throughout the move.

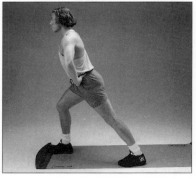

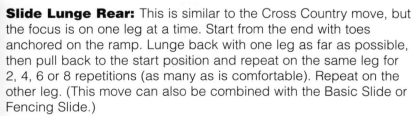

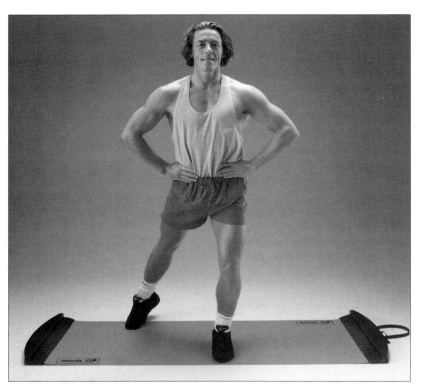

10. Speed Skate ◄

This move begins in the centre of the board in the athletic-ready stance. Push alternate legs out to the side and slightly to the rear. Return each foot to the centre position before pushing out the other leg.

Caution: Keep a check on your posture in this position. Sit back and don't lean forward from the waist. Don't hop or bounce, but ensure you slide the feet in and out. If your head is bobbing up and down, you are hopping (this is cheating!). Instead, keep the head level thoughout.

11. Low Profile Slide ►

This is the Basic Slide move performed in the athletic ready stance. It is performed at regular speed (4 counts) for the introductory and intermediate level and at double time (2 counts) for the advanced level.

Caution: Practise at the slower speed first and proceed with caution. Keep a check on your posture and ensure your head stays at the same height throughout. Don't let it bob up and down.

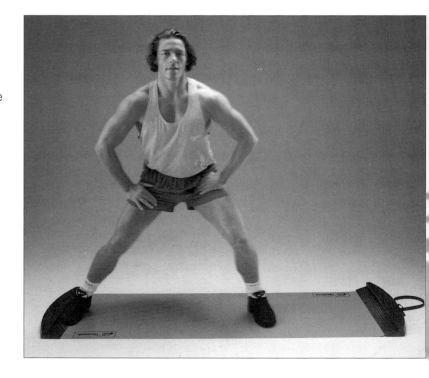

12. Slide Squat ►

Complete the Basic Slide, then move into the athletic ready stance. Stabilize your lead leg on the ramp, and go into a low squat, keeping the heels flat. Return to an upright position before pushing off again

Caution: As this is an advanced level move, practise it first at a slower speed.

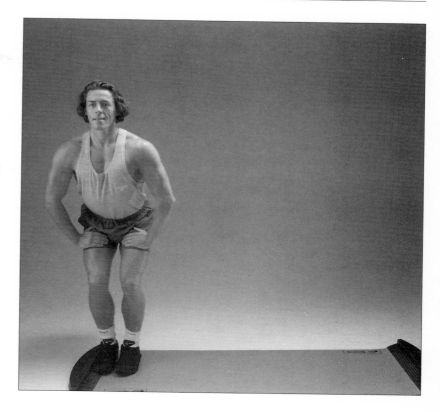

13. Slide Lift Single and Double ◄

Double: Complete the Basic Slide and, on contact with the ramp, raise up on to the toes of both feet. Make sure you maintain correct alignment as you raise.

Single: Complete the Basic Slide and, on contact with the ramp, raise up on to the toes of the lead leg and draw up the trail leg into a Leg or Knee Lift.

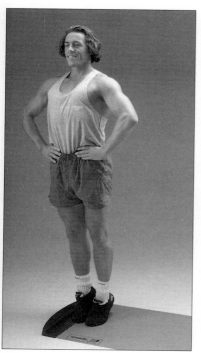

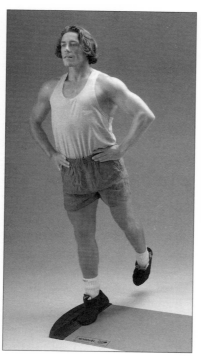

Far left: Slide Lift Double.
Left: Slide Lift Single.

14. Squat Pull

This move can be performed from any of the three start positions: from the front, from the end or from the centre. When you first practise this move, start from the end first, as this limits the depth of the squat, which is useful for beginners. Once you feel comfortable with this, the second stage is to start from the front with one foot stabilized on the ramp. The most advanced version is to start from the centre. Always start the Squat Pull from a stationary position.

Caution: Check your alignment constantly and take care not to over exert yourself.

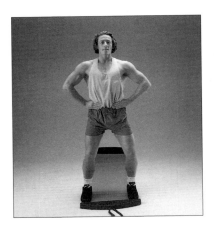
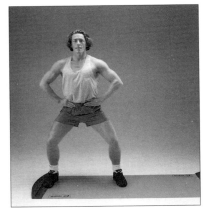
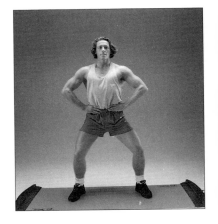

From the end: Stabilize both toes on the end ramp. Inch away from the ramp so the toes are just touching the edge. Slowly push both legs apart until the toes reach the edge of the board. Your knees are bent and aligned over the toes. Pull the legs back together and repeat 2, 3, 6 or 8 times (as many as is comfortable).

From the front: Stabilize one foot on the end ramp. Push out with the other leg until you are in a squat position. Check your alignment, then pull the leg back. Repeat 2, 4, 6 or 8 times as is comfortable.

From the centre: Slide to the centre of the board and face front in an upright position. Push the feet away from each other into a squat position. Check your alignment and pull the feet back together. Repeat as desired, but do not exceed 8 repetitions for the first few times.

15. Wide Slide

This is a modification of the Basic Slide. Start in the athletic ready stance. Push off and slide to the other end, but don't bring in the trail leg on recovery. Leave the trail leg out and push off again to the other side. It is performed at regular speed (4 counts) for the intermediate level and at double time (2 counts) for the advanced level.

Caution: Practise at the slower speed first and proceed with caution.

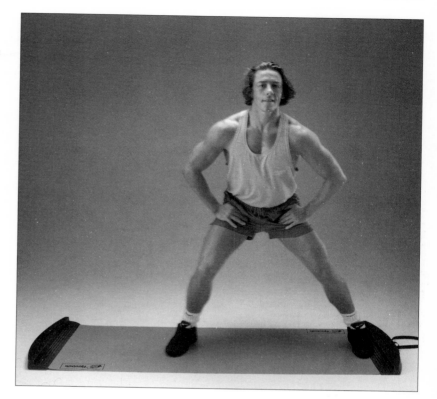

Putting It All Together

Once you have mastered all the moves, you need to put them together to give yourself a balanced workout. Remember, a workout should always follow this pattern: warm up, work out, cool down. You can substitute Slide Reebok for the aerobics section of the Basic Workout, or you can put your own programme together.

Slide Reebok can be done with or without music. If you use music you need to be sure that the music you choose is the right speed to enable you to complete the moves safely. The general music speeds for sliding range from 120 to 164 beats per minute but the recommended music speeds for this programme range from approximately 120 to 145 beats per minute. Beginners should always start at the lower end of the range.

Working with Music

If you choose to work out with music you can follow the Rhythmic Track Workout. All moves take four music beats to go from one end of the board to the other unless otherwise specified. The 'push off' and 'glide' phases take three counts in total and the 'recovery' phase takes place on the fourth count. Take care if you attempt any of the 'two count' slides as these are considerably faster (you will actually be travelling from side to side in one and a half beats). Make sure you have mastered the slower moves before you attempt the faster ones. The recommended speed for this introductory programme is 32 slides per minute.

Working without Music

If you choose to work out without music you can follow the Athletic Track Workout. Monitor your speed by counting the number of slides you do per minute. The recommended speed is 30 slides per minute. Maintain the rhythm by tuning in to your own comfort zone or listening to a loud clock ticking.

The Slide Reebok 30-minute Workout

Format	Approximate time
Warm-up and stretch	5 minutes
Slide aerobics workout	20 minutes
Cool-down and stretch	5 minutes

Warm-up and Stretch

Follow the warm-up instructions on page 122.

Slide Aerobics Workout

Choose either the Rhythmic Track or the Athletic Track Workout (see pages 135–136). As the Slide Reebok aerobics workout is the most demanding of all the programmes in this book, ensure you master all the entry levels before attempting either of these tracks, and make sure you stay within your training heart rate zone. For extra variety and challenge, you can add the following moves:

Slide Lunge Rear
Cross Country Wide
Speed Skate
Low Profile Slide (in 2 or 4 counts)
Slide Lift Single
Squat Pull
Wide Slide

Cool-down and Stretch

For the 30-minute workout, repeat the inner and outer thigh stretches from the warm-up, then turn to page 72 for the final stretch. If you wish to add a strengthening session, turn to page 66 and follow the cool-down instructions before doing any strengthening work. Always finish with the final stretch.

The Rhythmic Track Workout
(Entry Level 4)

Approximate time: 20 minutes
Music speed: 120–130 bpm

Move	No. of Slides
Basic Slide	32
Slide Touch Front	16
Slide Touch Rear	16
Basic Slide	16
Knee Lift Front	8
Knee Lift Across	8
Basic Slide	16
Knee Lift Front	8
Knee Lift Across	8
Basic Slide	16
Knee Lift Side	8
Hamstring Curl	8
Basic Slide	16
Knee Lift Side	8
Hamstring Curl	8
Basic Slide	16
Leg Lift Front	8
Leg Lift Rear	8
Basic Slide	16
Slide Lunge Side	16
Basic Slide	16
*Leg Lift Side	8

Move	No. of Slides
Basic Slide	8
Fencing Slide	8
Reverse Fencing Slide	16
*Slide Squat	8
Basic Slide	8
Cross Country Narrow	120
Basic Slide	16
*Slide Squat	8
Basic Slide	24
*Slide Lift Double	8
Basic Slide	24
Knee Lift Front	8
Knee Lift Across	8
Basic Slide	32
Knee Lift Side	8
Hamstring Curl	8
Basic Slide	16
*Leg Lift Side	8
Leg Lift Rear	8
Fencing Slide	16
Reverse Fencing Slide	16
Basic Slide	32

* Level 4 intensity moves, so proceed with caution.

Note: Always start and finish with the Basic Slide to gently ease in and out of your aerobics workout.

The Athletic Track Workout

(Entry Level 4)

Approximate time: 20 minutes

Move	No. of Slides	Move	No. of Slides
Basic Slide	30	**Basic Slide**	30
Slide Touch Front	15	***Slide Squat**	8
Slide Touch Rear	15	**Cross Country Narrow**	120
Knee Lift Front	15	**Basic Slide**	30
Knee Lift Across	15	**Slide Squat**	8
Basic Slide	30	**Basic Slide**	30
***Knee Lift Side**	15	***Slide Lift Double**	8
Hamstring Curl	15	**Basic Slide**	30
Basic Slide	30	**Slide Touch Front**	15
Leg Lift Front	15	**Slide Touch Rear**	15
Leg Lift Rear	15	**Basic Slide**	30
Basic Slide	30	**Knee Lift Front**	15
Slide Lunge Side	15	**Knee Lift Across**	15
***Leg Lift Side**	8	**Basic Slide**	15
Fencing Slide	15	**Knee Lift Side**	15
Reverse Fencing Slide	15	**Basic Slide**	15

* Level 4 intensity moves, so proceed with caution.

Note: Always start and finish with the Basic Slide to gently ease in and out of your aerobics workout.

Selecting a Health Club or Class

There are three main criteria to consider when selecting a club or class for the first time. The first is what type of exercise do you want to do and does that instructor or club cater for it? If not, what is on offer? Second, is the instructor professionally qualified and is the club or class run in a professional manner? The third question is how well do they treat their customers? Do they offer the standard of customer service you expect of professionals?

Qualifications

The RSA (Royal Society of Arts) certificate in exercise to music is the basic instructor qualification in the UK and is officially recognized by the Sports Council, along with the KFA (Keep Fit Association) certificate. To acquire the RSA certificate, instructors have to attend a minimum of 80 hours of tutor-based training and undertake an equal amount of home study. They have to sit both a theory and practical exam, which includes a thorough demonstration of teaching skills.

Qualifications are always being extended and developed, and NVQ (National Vocational Qualifications) will be introduced shortly in the UK along the lines of the European system. The current basic RSA certificate however is a good yardstick for measuring all other types of certificates and gives an insight into an instructor's experience.

In the USA there are two recognized qualifications, the ACE (American Council on Exercise – previously called IDEA) and AFAA (Aerobics and Fitness Association of America) certificates. Generally these take the form of self study, followed by a written paper and a brief, practical assessment of teaching skills.

When selecting an instructor you should check the number of years of teaching experience he/she has had and how often he/she attends workshops or conventions to keep abreast of the latest developments in fitness training. It's also worth checking if he/she has experience or qualifications in other related fields, such as physical therapy, dance or PE training, as this may extend the service on offer.

Customer Service

Having the right qualifications should ensure that the instructor you choose will be knowledgeable about his or her subject, but it is also important that you feel comfortable in his/her environment. So, before paying membership or class fees, find out as much as you can about the instructor or club in advance.

1. Ask friends, relatives, work colleagues if they attend a local club or class and what they feel about the place or people involved.
2. Telephone the instructor or club and find out what the procedure is for first-time attendees. Do ask to look around the club or watch a class before joining. All clubs should be keen to arrange an appointment and use the opportunity to sell a membership to you.
3. At your appointment with the instructor or club, check out the following:

Questions to ask an instructor

✦ What are his/her qualifications?
✦ How long has he/she been teaching?
✦ How many people are in the class and are the majority regulars? Have they been attending for a long time? Do many people drop out?
✦ Does he/she supply all the equipment or do you have to take your own?
✦ Is water available on the premises?
✦ Are showers available?
✦ Does he/she have a first-timer's policy or a particular class that would suit a beginner?

Points to consider

✦ Does he/she ask you about your exercise experience or your current level of activity?
✦ Does he/she ask you to complete a health questionnaire?
✦ Does he/she advise you to speak to your GP if you have any doubts about exercising?
✦ Is his/her manner welcoming?
✦ At the class, does he/she make you feel comfortable about joining in? Does he/she encourage you to wear the appropriate footwear for the impact exercises?
✦ Does he/she pay much attention to you? Does he/she watch how you perform and ensure you do the exercises safely?
✦ Does he/she give teaching tips throughout the exercises? And is time given for a thorough warm-up and cool-down?
✦ Does he/she encourage you to sip water when you need to?
✦ Does he/she ensure you can cope with the exercises and offer alternatives if necessary?
✦ Are you enjoying yourself – despite the sweat?

Questions to ask at the club

✦ What qualifications do the teaching staff have?
✦ What facilities are available to you and when for the membership category on offer?
✦ What extras do you have to pay for?
✦ Can you bring in guests and, if so, what is the extra cost?
✦ What is the policy for beginners? Are there beginners' classes or guided workouts within the gym area?
✦ Are there any first-aiders on site?

✦ What is the booking and cancellation procedure for classes or use of facilities?
✦ Does the club offer fitness assessments? When and where are these carried out? Is it somewhere private so that the whole club doesn't have to know your body-fat measurement or see that you can't reach your toes!
✦ How many members does the club have, and how many renew each year?
✦ Does the club offer trial periods, or will they give you a refund if you are not happy?

Points to consider

✦ Are you made to feel welcome the minute you walk through the door?
✦ Are the staff helpful and keen to answer all your questions and give you all the information you require?
✦ Do they ask about your health, current exercise experience and any particular interests you have?
✦ Do they insist that you fill in a health questionnaire and have a fitness assessment before being allowed to use any equipment?
✦ Do they insist that a customized exercise programme is worked out for you until you become familiar with the club and equipment?
✦ Do they offer advice on the most suitable classes for you to start off with?
✦ After you have joined the club, do the staff make an effort to remember your name? Are they still attentive to your needs? Do they ensure you get to hear about all the special offers or social events and encourage you to come along? Do they notice if you miss a class or don't attend for a while, and do they ask after your wellbeing?

Obviously the more positive a response you get from the instructor or club, the better the service they are likely to provide. If you don't get the information you want, ask to speak to another member of staff or try another instructor. And do let your instructor or club manager know if you are unhappy with your progress or the treatment you receive. If you politely inform them of any concerns or problems you may have, then you will at least give them the chance to put things right.

Maintaining Your Healthy Lifestyle

Taking up exercise on a regular basis is one step towards your new active way of life. Selecting a good environment in which to work out is crucial in encouraging you to continue with your exercise programme. But in order to maintain this new healthy lifestyle it's important that you are able to see ongoing results. Although exercise alone will make a certain amount of noticeable difference, for your body to gain optimum benefits from exercise it needs additional help. Exercise combined with other healthy living factors can make such a marked difference to how you look and feel that you won't want to fall back into your old habits at any cost.

Your eating and lifestyle habits and your personal outlook on life are all factors that contribute to your overall health and this chapter covers each of these aspects.

Healthy Eating

Health and fitness experts worldwide agree that a well-balanced diet, loaded with fresh, nutritious foods, combined with a regular and balanced regime of vigorous exercise is by far the best prescription for healthy living and good body maintenance.

However, busy lifestyles, limited time and funds, old habits, misconceptions and confusing media hype about the benefits or detriments of certain foodstuffs all contribute to hindering our success. But take heart! The first step is to understand a few basic facts about food and what it actually does for us.

The Excess Factor

All food provides energy, commonly known as calories. However, not all types of food can be usefully transformed within the body and unusable components of food are usually excreted. But certain types of food consumed in excess can end up being stored by the body as fat against a possible 'emergency' such as extreme levels of hunger or energy depletion. As starvation is a rare occurrence in the western world and energy depletion usually only happens in the case of endurance athletes, for many of us, eating too much food and not taking enough exercise can lead to weight problems.

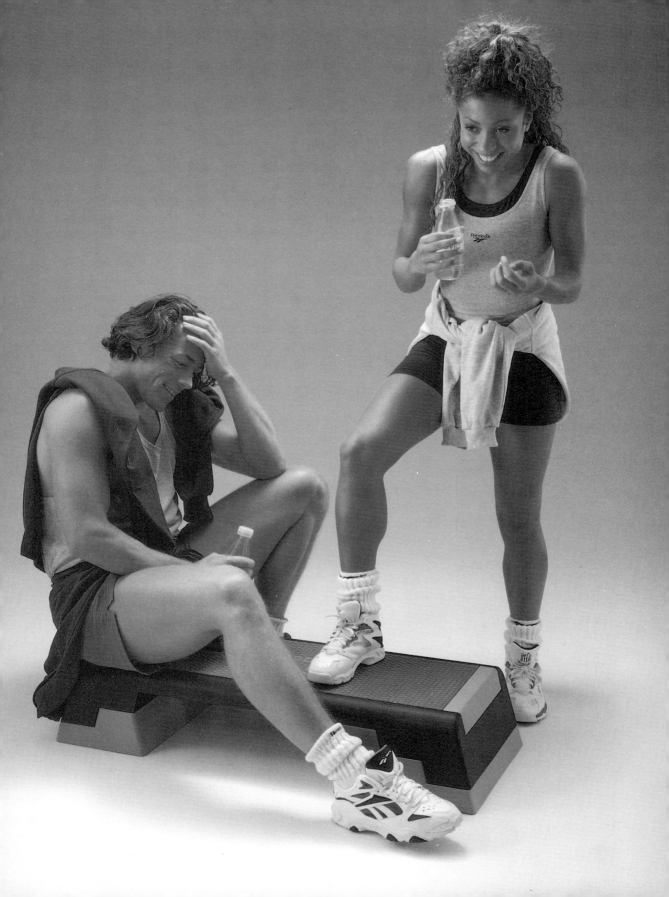

Some Facts About Food

✦ There is no such thing as 'good' food or 'bad' food. All foods carry some goodness, but fresh foods carry more than processed.

✦ No single food carries sufficient nutrients to completely nourish the body.

✦ Some types of food are superfluous to the body's requirements, e.g. processed sugar.

✦ Carbohydrates are not fattening.

✦ Fat is fattening.

✦ Most people underestimate the amount of fat they eat.

✦ Most people overestimate the amount of protein they need.

Food as Energy

The body needs a good supply of energy and nutrients in a form that it can use to help us maintain a healthy and energetic lifestyle and prevent illness.

There are six main food groups: vitamins, minerals, carbohydrate, fat, protein and water. The body requires a regular, balanced supply of the first five, plus approximately 1 litre of water per day in order to sustain itself.

Vitamins and Minerals

These are not a direct source of energy, but they do contribute to the proper functioning of the body. Vitamins and minerals interact closely with each other, by either helping or hindering a fellow vitamin or mineral to perform its function. A healthy balanced diet based on fresh whole foods should supply an adequate supply of all vitamins and minerals.

Carbohydrate, Fat and Protein

Each of these nutrients is broken down within the body and either stored for future use or used for rebuilding body tissue.

Sources of Carbohydrate

Complex Carbohydrates	Simple Carbohydrates
brown rice	fruit
pasta	fruit juice
potatoes	milk
parsnips	yogurt
pulses (legumes)	confectionary
bread	jam, preserves
breakfast cereals	puddings
flour, oats, millet, couscous, grains	pastries

Note: Although white bread, pasta and rice etc. are sources of complex carbohydrates, the whole-grain varieties offer greater fibre benefits and are generally considered more beneficial to health.

Carbohydrate

Carbohydrate is stored mainly as glycogen in the muscles and liver and used for short-term energy supplies. It is a good food source for all of us, but especially for athletes and the physically active as it is quickly transformed by the body into energy.

Carbohydrate should comprise 60–70 per cent of your total diet. A diet high in carbohydrate will ensure the body always has plenty of immediate energy supplies, both for everyday activities and for sport and exercise. A diet too low in carbohydrate will lead to early fatigue, particularly in active people. If carbohydrate is excluded as part of a weight-loss programme, as is often the case in low-calorie or crash dieting, the result will be a loss of muscle tissue rather than fat as the body turns to the muscles for its emergency energy stores.

Carbohydrates split into two groups: simple carbohydrates (sugary foods) and complex carbohydrates (starchy foods). In a healthy diet, it's the complex carbohydrates we need most, particularly the whole-grain versions, since these offer a greater fibre content, but beware of fatty accompaniments! The simple, sugary types of carbohydrate do offer some nutritional value, especially if sourced from natural food products such as fruit, milk or natural yogurt. Where possible, however, try to cut down on your intake of foods such as cakes, confectionary and biscuits since these contain both fat and sugar and, do not offer the same level of nutritional value.

When planning your diet, therefore aim to make up the majority of your carbohydrate intake from the complex types. For a healthy nutritional package, think of whole-grain starches (such as pasta, rice and potatoes) and natural sugars (such as from fruit) for necessary energy, and refined sugars for unnecessary energy but maybe an occasional indulgence.

Fat

Fat is stored as fat tissue around the internal organs, within the muscles and under the skin and is used as a long-term energy store. Fat consumption should be kept to a minimum, especially in the case of inactive people. Fat takes longer than carbohydrate to be transformed into energy, and excess fat soon builds up around the body and can lead to overweight and health problems such as heart disease and abnormal blood pressure. However, a certain amount of fat is important in the diet as it is a valuable source of essential fatty acids and the fat-soluble vitamins A, D, E. and K. More importantly, it is required for its protective and insulation factors and for the crucial role it plays in the proper functioning of the female hormones.

The visible fats	Low-fat alternatives
Butter, margarine	Low-fat spread
Fatty meat	Lean cuts, skinless chicken, turkey
Hard and soft cheese	Low-fat cheeses or cottage cheese, fromage frais

The hidden fats	Low-fat alternatives
Cheese sauces	Use low-fat cheese or limit the portion
Creamy pasta sauces	Tomato or vegetable sauces
Full-fat milk and yogurts	Skimmed milk and low-fat yogurts
Crisps, cheesy-type snacks and salted peanuts	Dried or fresh fruit, raw vegetables
Garlic bread	Make your own with low-fat spread, fresh garlic and a French stick
Chocolate, chocolate products	Fresh fruit
Sweet pies and pastries	Fresh-fruit desserts
Processed meats	Low-fat versions, fish pâté or limit the portion
Ready-made meals	Low-fat versions

Tips for Lowering Your Fat Intake

Aim to reduce your daily intake of fat to 20 to 30 per cent of your total diet. You can do this in some of the following ways:

+ Choose low-fat alternatives.
+ Check for the 'hidden' fat content in ready-made or processed foods.
+ Trim the fat off meat and remove the skin from chicken before cooking.
+ Don't coat foods heavily in oil, butter or lard when cooking.
+ Use cheese in moderation, especially in cooking, as many brands contain a high level of fat.
+ Steam, grill or bake rather than fry foods.
+ Use covered pots for baking and reduce the amount of oil when basting joints.

A woman whose body fat becomes too low – a common occurrence in female athletes and ballet dancers – may stop menstruating. While this problem can be rapidly remedied by an adjustment to the individual's diet and exercise schedule, it can still have long-term implications such as increased risk of osteoporosis.

Generally, it's considered healthier to choose vegetable fats in preference to animal fats as the latter are made up mostly of unsaturated fat. However, all fats should be consumed with moderation. It's worth checking the labels on all products to see exactly how much fat is included. Often the levels of fat are not obvious in ready-made or canned foods, and these are what is known as the 'hidden' fats.

Protein

Protein is normally used for rebuilding muscle and body tissue but can also be used for emergency supplies of energy when carbohydrate stores are depleted, for instance towards the end of a long-duration, high-intensity exercise period.

Protein is vital for growth and reconstruction purposes, but its role is often overestimated and misunderstood. Many people assume that eating more protein will make them stronger or bigger – it won't. The body can only usefully use a certain amount and, although excess protein is excreted by the body, very high intakes can put undue strain on the liver and kidneys. Additionally, part of the excess protein may be stored as fat, an equally unwelcome prospect. Protein should comprise only 12–15 per cent of your total diet.

What Should We Eat?

Good Sources of Protein

beans

fish

lean meat

lentils

liver

milk, cheese and yogurt

nuts and seeds

peas

poultry

A balanced, healthy diet should be high in fresh fruit and vegetables, high in whole grains such as brown rice, bread and pasta, moderate in meat and fish, and limited in the fats and sugars. Plan your meals to fit in with the recommended guidelines below. Cook with care and shop selectively. Scrutinize the packaging of foods to check for hidden fats, sugar and salt as well as artificial additives.

How Much Should We Eat?

A balanced, healthy diet for an active person should be made up of:

+ 60–70 per cent carbohydrate
+ 20–30 per cent fat (at least 50 per cent of this should be unsaturated)
+ 12–15 per cent protein
+ Plus an adequate supply of vitamins and minerals from a wholesome diet.

* 'Foods, Nutrition and Sports Performance'. *Journal of Sports Sciences*, 1991.

Check Your Eating Habits

To start yourself off on your new eating plan, keep a record of everything you eat, using the chart in the appendix, and calculate the proportion of carbohydrate, fat and protein in your diet.

Make a note of any adjustments you need to make before you plan your next food shopping trip.

Eating and Exercise for Weight Loss

It is now agreed that sensible eating together with exercise is the best formula for improving health and controlling weight.

The reasons are twofold. First, exercise burns calories and speeds up the metabolism (the rate at which our bodies burn up the energy from food). Second, the more we exercise and the more muscle tone we develop, the more calories we burn up.

Dieting without Exercise

Most weight problems occur from an imbalance in energy input and output. In other words, someone who eats more calories (energy) than he/she needs will put on weight, usually in the form of fat.

For long-term weight loss it is not enough merely to reduce our food intake without increasing our level of activity. Remember, the body is a very adaptable machine. So, if its regular supply of energy is reduced, it will automatically switch into self-preservation mode, causing the metabolism to slow down so that the body burns much less energy.

If we continue to eat less for a period of time without increasing our activity level, the body looks for other sources of energy which are not currently being used. Therefore, if the skeletal muscles are not being used regularly, the body will 'dip' into these for its 'emergency' supply. However, once normal eating habits are resumed and if exercise is still excluded, the body will be more prone to a build-up of fat, since no demands are being placed on the muscles.

Dieting with Exercise

On the other hand, if we reduce our calorie intake and ensure that the calories consumed are 'quality' calories from a diet high in carbohydrates (the type the body can use quickly), and at the same time increase our activity level (energy output), we are more likely to achieve a healthy, lean, toned body. And a lean, toned body burns more calories.

One of the best forms of exercise for weight loss is aerobic exercise as this specifically uses fat and carbohydrate as its energy source. This is why the experts recommend specific bouts of aerobic exercise at a specific intensity for a specific length of time. Not only does this offer cardiovascular benefits, but it also ensures that the body's energy-burning system can make use of the stored supplies of glycogen (from carbohydrate) and fat.

For best results, combine aerobic exercise with resistance exercise. Resistance exercise increases our muscle mass, and the more muscle mass we have, the more calories we will burn.

Healthy-eating Tips

+ Eat little and often rather than starving all day and bingeing at night.

+ Don't buy high-fat or sugary snacks you can't resist.

+ Keep healthy, easy-to-nibble snacks around the house such as dried fruit, fresh fruit and carrot straws to help you through those moments of weakness.

+ Drink plenty of fresh water – it cleanses the system and is great for the skin.

+ Always eat breakfast – it's the most important meal of the day and provides essential energy. Make sure it's a high-carbohydrate, low-fat breakfast.

+ Don't skip lunch or eat on the run. Even if you only take half an hour, sit down and enjoy a whole-meal sandwich some yogurt and fruit and a glass of mineral water.

Smoking and Health

It is well known that smoking can increase our risk of respiratory disease, coronary heart disease and certain cancers, and the dangers of passive smoking (inhaling smoke from other people's cigarettes) are now well documented. However, from a nutritional perspective, smoking depletes the body's vitamins and mineral levels, thus weakening the immune system and making the body more prone to disease.

Smoking and Exercise

Smoking is a difficult habit to break, but there are now many products, methods and support groups available to help even the most committed of smokers give up.

Often underestimated are the benefits of regular exercise in helping to kick the smoking habit. Aerobic exercise, in particular, appears to have been successful for some. It is thought that the anti-stress benefits from increased activity and the increased adrenalin levels that are instigated by exercise may have something to do with making the smoker feel less like smoking. However, be sure to inform your fitness instructor or club of your smoking habits before taking up a new exercise programme.

Social and Emotional Health

A high level of stress and negative personal outlook on life are attributed to many health problems. While regular exercise can be a great antidote to stress – particularly the type of exercise that demands your full attention, as this gives the brain some 'time off' from daily worries – it's all too easy to fall into the 'exercise is the answer to everything' trap.

Exercise is ideal for diverting the mind, releasing pent-up anger, relaxation, improving self-image and self-confidence and for 'taking time out'. In addition, exercise – particularly longer bouts of aerobic exercise – appears to induce a 'feel-good' factor either during or after the session. But it's equally important to realize that 'torturing' yourself by attempting to squeeze in frequent bouts of exercise on top of an already hectic and stressful lifestyle will only add to the existing stress, fatigue and associated health problems. The only answer is to review your lifestyle and reassess your priorities to bring life back on to an even keel.

Stress – the Secret Enemy

The body is well equipped to cope with a certain amount of stress. When placed under stress the body increases its output of adrenalin, which allows the body to react swiftly to potentially dangerous situations. However, in today's society, increased pressure to perform to high standards, job insecurity and economic pressure all contribute to producing increased stress levels in adults and youngsters alike.

Since stress is now so commonplace, we don't always realize the extent of the damage it may be causing. Furthermore, because stress can be difficult to measure, it's sometimes not taken seriously as a genuine cause of distress or illness. And an overworked individual may be reluctant to take time off for stress-related illnesses for fear of being made to feel that he or she is 'falling down' on the job. It is therefore important to familiarize yourself with your own 'coping levels' of stress and decide on a healthy cut-off point.

Stress-related Ailments

Some illnesses can be brought on or heightened by undue stress. These include migraine, certain allergies, neck, shoulder or back pain, digestive problems and circulation problems.

Use the chart below to help assess your current stress level and determine what action you can take to build a more balanced lifestyle.

If you recognize any of these signs, you may well be suffering from too much stress. Stop and take stock of your lifestyle.

Six Steps to Recognizing and Managing Stress

1. Take note of your reactions in times of stress. It is most likely you will react the same way each time. By noting your reactions, you can monitor the situations or people that cause your to react in this way and learn to handle or avoid them.
2. The body has certain physiological reactions to stress, for example, rapid shallow breathing, quickening of the heartbeat, sweating, tensing of the muscles. Again, note if and when any of these happen to you to help you manage the stressful situation.
3. Review the recent events in your life. Certain events are considered more stressful than others (see below), or a build-up of minor events may add up to sleepless nights or irritability.
4. Write down all the aspects of your life that you are currently finding stressful. Then list all the possible solutions — even the ones you don't like the idea of at first or that seem ridiculous. Once you have focused on the problem you will more than likely find the answer.
5. Don't be afraid to seek help if you feel you can't tackle your problems alone. Stewing over them will make you more stressed out.
6. Manage the stress. Now that you have recognized how you react in times of stress and identified at least some of the causes, use the stress management techniques described on page 148.

Typical Stressful Life Events

Death of family member, close friend or pet
Divorce or breakdown of relationship
Parents' divorce
Ageing parents
Serious injury or illness
Ill health of family member
Moving house
Getting married (especially for women)
Sexual problems with partner
Pregnancy
Changing job
Redundancy
Increased workload
Trouble with workmates or superiors
Exams, tests, or work evaluation.

Recognize Your Stress Level

Note which of the following typical signs of stress you find yourself doing and ask yourself what or who is the cause:

Wringing hands

Fidgeting with hair, clothes or object

Laughing, giggling excessively

Blinking, twitching or incessant coughing

Unable to sit still for a length of time

Sleepless nights

Compulsive eating

Not eating

Drinking too much alcohol

Frequent loss of temper

Unreasonable loss of temper

Shouting a lot

Constant feelings of anger or frustration

Depression

Bursting into tears easily or for no apparent reason

Jumping up when certain people enter the room

Finishing sentences midway.

Your Personal Outlook

People react to and handle stress in different ways. Those who are content and self-confident are usually better able to put life in perspective and manage the more stressful parts of their lives. They are also likely to recover more quickly from extreme situations such as bereavement or grief

Personal outlook can also have an effect on stress levels. Those who believe their happiness is someone else's responsibility and who always blame others for their misfortunes are likely to find certain situations more stressful than those who believe they are responsible for their own happiness and who are in control of their lives.

Detecting and managing the stress in your life is key to enjoying a healthy lifestyle. Exercise will certainly help, but it is not the whole solution.

Stress-management Techniques

Having identified an unpleasant level of stress in your life, the ideal solution is to remove the stressful factor completely from your life. However, this is not always practical or realistic, and some stresses such as exams, heavy work projects with specific deadlines or, indeed, grief and bereavement, have to be lived through. The method of managing stress depends in the first place on the nature of the stress.

Anger-based Stress

This can be very self-destructive if turned inward or bottled up. Anger in itself is a perfectly natural reaction and usually an instigator of change. Everybody should feel free to express anger when warranted, but frequent outbursts signify underlying problems that need to be looked into further.

Suggested Action

Try vigorous exercise, either a thrash about on the squash court, a long run or walk, an aerobics class or workout in the gym. Many people find they play or work out well when angry, but beware of injuring yourself in the heat of the moment. Equally, this may only prove to be a temporary relief, since the cause of the anger will still have to be dealt with, especially the cause of frequent anger.

Grief-based Stress

Grief is often associated with bereavement, but it can also be caused by major life changes such as marriage or relationship break-ups, moving house or changing jobs.

Suggested Action

This is a time for nurturing and comfort and not to be too self-critical. Be kind to yourself. Take long warm baths, gentle stretch and tone classes, yoga, long walks in the fresh air, massages, or simply wrap yourself in a blanket and watch your favourite movies in the privacy of your own home where you can sob or smile as suits you. Ask friends and family for support and understanding. 'Comforting' is an important factor in grief-based stress management, but it won't solve the problem, only the symptoms. Be prepared to ask for professional help with symptoms that won't go away.

Depression-based Stress

Depression is often repressed anger that expresses itself in lethargy and 'heavy' feelings. Exercise can sometimes help lift depression, while at other times it can make it seem worse, as it may lead to poor performance in your sport or exercise regime, and thus add to your feelings of self-dislike.

Suggested Action

Try sports that divert the mind or social activities such as class workouts, running groups, walking groups or dancing. In particular, choose the activities you are good at. This is not the time to attempt an activity you've always found difficult. If depression lingers or the cause is not clear, check it out with a professional counsellor.

Anxiety-based Stress

This is not always the obvious kind of stress that we associate with rushing about and having too much to do. Instead, it's the type that can creep up on you insidiously over a period of time, leading to very subtle, sometimes imperceptible, symptoms.

Suggested Action

Take plenty of exercise and fresh air, long walks, cycling, running, stretch or aerobics classes, yoga or meditation, or just sit quietly. Take time out on your own, doing things for yourself to increase your sense of self-worth.

Total Health

Although exercise and diet are vital for taking care of the mechanical aspects of physical health, the health of the mind is just as important. To be truly healthy, it's important to give time to both the physical and emotional sides of your life. How often do you do something creative or productive that gives you a tremendous feeling of self-satisfaction? This could be anything from painting a picture to weeding the garden. Creativity and productivity are good for the soul and for building self-esteem. When we feel good about ourselves it's much easier to feel generous towards others.

Time is precious, and time spent exercising and improving your health and wellbeing, whether training for a marathon or walking the dog, is time well spent because it's *your* time – time you have chosen to invest in yourself that will pay incomparable dividends. It is important that you enjoy every minute of your exercise programme and that you receive the best coaching and encouragement available. Follow the guidelines in this book, and you should learn how to exercise regularly, safely and enjoyably and how to develop your exercise programme as your skills and fitness levels improve.

Fill your life with activities, events and behaviour that you can enjoy and be proud of. Don't forget the creative aspects as well as the day-to-day survival aspects.

To be truly fit and healthy, exercise that body, feed it good fuel, fuel your creative mind, watch those stress levels, but most importantly, live life to the full and remember 'life is not a spectator sport!'

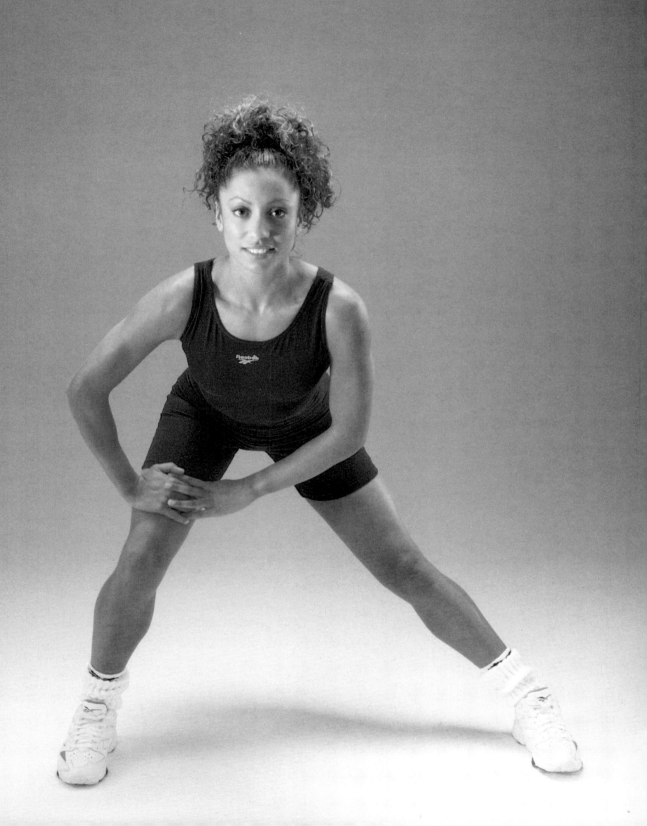

Appendix

Progress Chart 1:
Personal Measurements

	Week 1 Date:	Week 6 Date:	Inches (cm) lost or gained
Chest/bust	inches (cm)	inches (cm)	
Upper arms	inches (cm)	inches (cm)	
Waist	inches (cm)	inches (cm)	
Hips	inches (cm)	inches (cm)	
Thighs	inches (cm)	inches (cm)	
Calves	inches (cm)	inches (cm)	

How to Use this Chart
1. Measure yourself on the first day of your new healthy lifestyle.
2. Only measure yourself once on the prescribed weeks.
3. Note down *all* the changes – both losses and gains.
4. Use to keep yourself on track with your new regime.

Progress Chart 2:
Personal Performance

Test	Week 1 Date:	Week 6 Date:	Comments
Aerobic fitness			
Hip flexors (knee of extended leg should not bend)			
Hamstrings (raised leg vertical)			
Quadriceps (heel on buttocks)			
Soleus (ball of foot two fingers- width from platform)			
Abdominal strength (lift and hold for 10 counts or more)			

How to Use this Chart

1. Follow the tests on pages 39–3.

2. Rate yourself according to your performance, using the guidelines below:

0 = better than the test 1 = meets the test criteria 2 = almost there 3 = getting there 4 = struggling 5 = poor

3. Repeat the tests on Week 6 and enter your new scores.

4. Use these scores to see how far you have progressed and to plan the focus for your exercise programme. For example, if you score only 4s and 5s on flexibility, then you need to ensure you include plenty of stretching and mobility work in your exercise schedule.

Progress Chart 3:
Check Your Eating Habits

Week No:
Date:

Target Daily Calories:

	Mon	Tues	Wed	Thurs	Fri	Sat	Sun
Breakfast							
Elevenses							
Lunch							
Tea break							
Evening meal							
Snacks/Nibbles							
Total estimated calories							

Target Food Ratios
Carbohydrates: 60–70 per cent
Fat: 20–30 per cent
Protein: 12–15 per cent

How to Use this Chart
1. It's very easy to forget what we've eaten in a day, let alone in a week. In order to get a clear picture of your eating habits, note down *everything* you eat throughout the day.
2. Once you have charted your eating habits for a few days you will soon see the changes you need to make. Decide on your target calories per day and plan your diet accordingly. Remember to aim for that healthy combination of carbohydrate, fat and protein.
3. Try to develop a new eating style and keep this chart handy and complete it again a few weeks into your new eating plan so that you can compare the difference.

Progress Chart 4:
Weekly Exercise Schedule

Date:

Week No:	Monday	Tuesday	Wednesday	Thursday
Activity				
How long				
How hard				
How far (running, walking, etc.)				

	Target	Actual
Total hours of exercise per week:		
Total number of rest days:		
Total number of calories used:		
Total number of calories eaten:		
Calorie balance:		

Targets for next week:

Friday	Saturday	Sunday	Totals

How to Use this Chart

1. Enter the activity, and how long and how hard you exercised (and, if appropriate, how far). If you did not undertake any activity on a particular day, enter rest day.

2. Use the guidelines on page 157 to calculate the total number of hours and rest days, and the total number of calories used. Compare your results with your targets.

3. Use this chart to keep an ongoing record of your progress and estimate your exercise targets for the following week.

Progress Chart 5:
Weekly Walking Log

Date:

Week No

Goal	Day	Exercise Pulse	Recovery Pulse	Walk Reebok Workout	Total Time and Distance
	Sunday				
	Monday				
	Tuesday				
	Wednesday				
	Thursday				
	Friday				
	Saturday				
Target Heart Rate		**To**		**Weekly Total**	

Calorie Expenditure Guidelines

Below are three charts based on the energy expenditure of the three Reebok University programmes. Select the body weight nearest to your own to give you an approximate guide to your own energy expenditure.

Energy Expenditure by Body Weight for Reebok University Programmes

(approximate kcals by body weight)

Step Reebok® Performing Basic Step, without arm movements, on a 6 inch platform

	8 stone 51 kg	9 stone 57 kg	10 stone 63.5 kg	11 stone 70 kg	12 stone 76 kg
30 mins	153	171	189	110	228
60 mins	306	342	378	420	456

Slide Reebok™ On a 6 foot board at a speed of 120 bpm

	8 stone 51 kg	9 stone 57 kg	10 stone 63.5 kg	11 stone 70 kg	12 stone 76 kg
30 mins	160	180	200	220	240
60 mins	321	359	400	441	479

Walk Reebok (and the Basic Workout)

	8 stone 61 kg	9 stone 57 kg	10 stone 63.5 kg	11 stone 70 kg	12 stone 76 kg
30 mins	100	111	124	137	148
60 mins	199	222	248	273	296

These figures have been based on energy expenditure studies of the three activities. The Basic Workout is a generic type of activity, and while a few studies have been carried out on similar types of low- and high-impact aerobics it would be misleading to give calorific guidelines on activities that are not identical. However, generally, low-impact aerobics (e.g. the Basic Workout) is estimated to have about the same calorific expenditure value as walking.

Bibliography and Further Reading

Aerobics Instructor Manual. ACE (American Council on Exercise), USA, 1993.

Allied Dunbar National Fitness Survey. The Sports Council and The Health Education Authority, UK, 1992. (Summary available from the Sports Council.)

Bean, Anita. *The Complete Guide to Sports Nutrition.* A & C Black, UK, 1993.

Bevan, James. *A Pictorial Handbook of Anatomy and Physiology.* Mitchell Beazley, UK, 1978.

Cross, Mervyn, Gibbs, Nathan, and Gray, James. *The Sporting Body.* McGraw Hill, Australia, 1991.

Cullum, Rodney and Mowbray, Lesley. *The English YMCA Guide to Exercise to Music* (new revised edn). Pelham Books, UK, 1992.

Egger, Garry and Champion, Nigel. *The Fitness Leaders' Handbook.* Kangaroo Press, Australia, 1985.

Foods, Nutrition and Sports Performance. Journal of Sports Sciences, UK, 1991.

Francis, Peter and Lorna. *If It Hurts, Don't Do It.* Prima Publishing and Communications Ltd, USA, 1988.

Kusinitz, Ivan and Fine, Morton. *Your Guide to Getting Fit* (2nd edn). Mayfield Publishing Co., USA, 1991.

McArdle, William D., Katch, Frank I. and Victor L. *Exercise Physiology, Energy, Nutrition and Human Performance.* Lea & Febiger, USA, 1991.

May, Jill. *A Reference Manual for Teachers of Dance Exercise.* W. Foulsham & Co. Ltd, UK, 1988.

Moran, Diana and Franks, Helen. *Bone Boosters.* Boxtree, UK, 1993.

Norris, Christopher M. *Sports Injuries: Diagnosis and Management for Physiotherapists.* Butterworth, UK, 1993.

Physical Education Association. *New Directions in Physical Education* (vol. 2, ed. Neil Armstrong). Human Kinetics, UK, 1992.

Rowett, H. G. K. *Basic Anatomy and Physiology* (2nd edn). John Murray Ltd, UK, 1983.

Slide Reebok Instructor Manual. Reebok University Publications.

Step Reebok Instructor Manual. Reebok University Publications.

Thompson, C. W. *Manual of Structural Kinesiology* (9th edn). C. V. Mosby Co., USA, 1981.

Walk Reebok Instructor Manual. Reebok University Publications.

Wirhed, Rolf. *Athletic Ability and the Anatomy of Motion.* Harpoon Publications, Sweden, 1984.

Useful Addresses

In the UK

The Exercise Association of England Ltd
Unit 4, Angel Gate, 326 City Road, London
EC1V 2PT
Tel: 0171 278 0811
(Information on safe and effective exercise
and on finding a qualified teacher in your
area)

The Sports Council
16 Upper Woburn Place, London
WC1H OQP
Tel: 0171 388 1277
(Information on sporting and exercise organizations)

The Central Council for Physical Recreation
Francis House, Francis Street, London
SW1 1DE
Tel: 0171 828 3163
(Information on dance, movement and fitness organizations)

The Health Education Authority
Hamilton House, Mabledon Place, London
WC1H 9TX
Tel: 0171 383 3833
(Advice on general health matters)

The British Heart Foundation
14 Fitzhardinge Street, London W1H 4DH
Tel: 0171 935 0815
(Advice on preventing heart disease)

The British Nutrition Foundation
High Holborn House, 52-54 High Holborn,
London WC1V 6RQ
Tel: 0171 404 6504
(Advice on healthy eating)

The National Osteoporosis Society
PO Box 10, Radstock, Bath BA3 3YB
Tel: 0171 388 1277
(Advice on preventing osteoporosis)

The British School of Osteopathy
1-4 Suffolk Street, London SW1Y 4HQ
Tel: 0171 930 9254
(Advice on finding a registered osteopath)

In the USA

ACE (American Council on Exercise)
PO Box 910449, San Diego, CA 92191

AFAA (Aerobics and Fitness Association of
America)
15250 Ventura Blvd, Suite 200, Sherman
Oaks, CA 91403

ACSM (American College of Sports
Medicine)
PO Box 1440, Indianapolis, IN 46206

IDEA (International Association of Fitness
Professionals)
6190 Cornerstone Court East, Suite 204, San
Diego, CA 92121

Muscle Mixes Music
PO Box 533967, Orlando, FL 32853
Tel: (001) 407 872 7576

The Author

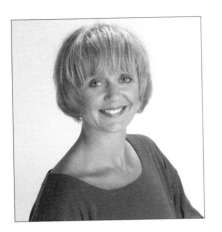

Five years running her own fitness company and instructor training courses, followed by eight years with Reebok in marketing and educational development has established Chantal Gosselin as a prime mover in the fitness industry. Responsible for the UK launch of the Step Reebok, Walk Reebok and Slide Reebok programmes as well as the UK National Aerobics Championships and the first-ever nationwide fitness roadshow, she also recently hosted and directed the European Aerobics Championships.

A founder member of the development team for the Physical Education Health and Exercise Certificate in the UK, Chantal has recently been elected as Vice Chair of the Exercise Association of England, the new national governing body for exercise. Chantal has a BA in Performance Arts and a postgraduate certificate of education from London University. She is a member of the American College of Sports Medicine (ACSM), IDEA, the American Alliance for Health, Physical Education, Recreation and Dance (AAHPERD), the Aerobics and Fitness Association of American (AFAA) and the Chartered Institute of Marketing.

Chantal has developed and led the UK Reebok University team to its current unrivalled status and continues to be retained by Reebok UK as a Fitness Development Consultant.

Reebok University Classes

Many instructors around the world have been trained by Reebok to teach safe and effective classes in all the Reebok University programmes. For details of your local Reebok University class or one-to-one training at home from a trained Reebok instructor, ring the hotline number:
01494 816666